Comprehensive
Aquatic Therapy

Comprehensive Aquatic Therapy

Edited by

Bruce E. Becker, M.D.

Assistant Professor of Physical Medicine and Rehabilitation,
Wayne State University School of Medicine, Detroit; Vice President
of Medical Affairs, Rehabilitation Institute of Michigan, Detroit

Andrew J. Cole, M.D.

Puget Sound Sports and Spine Physicians, Bellevue, Washington;
Medical Director, Overlake Hospital Medical Center, Spine Center,
Bellevue; Clinical Assistant Professor of Physical Medicine and
Rehabilitation, Department of Physical Therapy, University of Texas
Southwestern Medical Center, Dallas

With 13 Contributing Authors

Butterworth–Heinemann
Boston   Oxford   Johannesburg   Melbourne   New Delhi   Singapore

Every effort has been made to ensure that the drug dosage schedules within this text are accurate and conform to standards accepted at time of publication. However, as treatment recommendations vary in the light of continuing research and clinical experience, the reader is advised to verify drug dosage schedules herein with information found on product information sheets. This is especially true in cases of new or infrequently used drugs.

∞ Recognizing the importance of preserving what has been written, Butterworth–Heinemann prints its books on acid-free paper whenever possible.

AMERICAN FORESTS
GLOBAL RELEAF 2000   Butterworth–Heinemann supports the efforts of American Forests and the Global ReLeaf program in its campaign for the betterment of trees, forests, and our environment.

Library of Congress Cataloging-in-Publication Data
Comprehensive aquatic therapy / edited by Bruce E. Becker, Andrew J. Cole.
    p.   cm.
    Includes bibliographical references and index.
    ISBN 0-7506-9649-4
    1. Hydrotherapy. I. Becker, Bruce E. II. Cole, Andrew J.
    [DNLM: 1. Hydrotherapy. 2. Rehabilitation--methods. WB 520 C737 1997]
    RM811.C675 1997
    615.8'53--dc21
    DNLM/DLC
    for Library of Congress   97-12662
                                                           CIP

British Library Cataloguing-in-Publication Data
A catalogue record for this book is available from the British Library.

The publisher offers special discounts on bulk orders of this book.
For information, please contact:

Manager of Special Sales
Butterworth–Heinemann
313 Washington Street
Newton, MA 02158-1626
Tel: 617-928-2500
Fax: 617-928-2620

For information on all Butterworth–Heinemann publications available, contact our World Wide Web home page at: http://www.bh.com/

10 9 8 7 6 5 4 3 2 1

Printed in the United States of America

To my friend and wife Carol, whose example in time management has made this book possible, and whose support has given it direction; to her parents Charles and Mildred Wedemeyer, whose dedication to academic excellence provided motivation; to my children Adrianne and Derek, for their forbearance and love; and to my dad Erhart Becker, who inspires effort and goodwill in our entire family. I deeply regret that my mother did not live to see this publication, but believe that her spirit will assist sales.

B.E.B.

To my grandmother, Anne Shulman, whose vision spanned generations and whose love and enthusiasm brought generations together; my wife, Carolyn Adams Cole, without whose love all else would lose meaning; and my daughter, Anne Adams Cole, in whom all my hopes are embodied.

A.J.C.

Contents

Contributing Authors

Claudio Gil Soares de Araújo, M.D., Ph.D.
Medical Director, Clinica de Medicina do Exercíco, Rio de Janeiro, Brazil; Medical Director, Cardiac Rehabilitation Program, Hospital Universitario Clementino Fraga Filho–Universidade Federal do Rio de Janeiro; Associate Professor of Physiology, Universidade Federal Fluminense, Rio de Janeiro

Oded Bar-Or, M.D.
Professor of Pediatrics, McMaster University Faculty of Health Sciences, Hamilton, Ontario, Canada; Director, Children's Exercise and Nutrition Centre, Department of Pediatrics, Hamilton Health Sciences Corporation, Chedoke Division

Bruce E. Becker, M.D.
Assistant Professor of Physical Medicine and Rehabilitation, Wayne State University School of Medicine, Detroit; Vice President of Medical Affairs, Rehabilitation Institute of Michigan, Detroit

David K. Brennan, M.Ed.
Assistant Professor of Physical Medicine and Rehabilitation, Baylor College of Medicine, Houston; Coordinator, Aquatic Rehabilitation, Medifit Human Performance Center, Houston

Andrew J. Cole, M.D.
Puget Sound Sports and Spine Physicians, Bellevue, Washington; Medical Director, Overlake Hospital Medical Center, Spine Center, Bellevue; Clinical Assistant Professor of Physical Medicine and Rehabilitation, Department of Physical Therapy, University of Texas Southwestern Medical Center, Dallas

Jill Napoletan Craig, M.S.
Independent Research Physiologist and Coordinator, Austin, Texas; Sports Medicine Consultant, The Hills Fitness Center, Austin; Faculty, Department of Health and Kinesiology, Austin Community College, Austin

Jonathan Paul De Vierville, Ph.D., M.S.W., L.M.S.W.-A.C.P., L.P.C., T.R.M.T.
Associate Professor of History and The Humanities, Department of Social and Behavioral Sciences, St. Philip's College, San Antonio; Director, Alamo Plaza Spa at the Menger Hotel, San Antonio

Richard A. Eagleston, M.A., P.T., A.T.C.
S.T.A.R. Physical Therapy, Redwood City, California

Gwendolyn Garrett, M.A., OTR
Director of Ambulatory Services, Rehabilitation Management, Inc., Richmond, Virginia; President, Aquatic Rehabilitation Consultants, Smithfield, Virginia

Juliana Larson, B.S., L.M.T.
Instructor of Hydrotherapy and Massage, Massage Department, Lane Community College and Cascade Massage Institute, Eugene, Oregon; Aquatic Supervisor, Sheldon Pool and Fitness Center, Eugene

David M. Morris, M.S., P.T.
Associate Professor of Physical Therapy, University of Alabama at Birmingham

Marilou Moschetti, B.Sc., P.T.A.
Executive Director, AquaTechnics Consulting Group, Aptos, California; Aquatic Physical Therapy Coordinator, Wellness and Rehabilitation Center, Watsonville Community Hospital

Richard G. Ruoti, Ph.D., P.T., C.S.C.S.
Clinical Operations Director, NovaCare, Inc., Warminster, Pennsylvania

Steven A. Stratton, Ph.D., P.T., A.T.C.
President, Alamo Physical Therapy Inc., San Antonio; Clinical Associate Professor of Physical Medicine and Rehabilitation, Physical Therapy Department, University of Texas Health Science Center at San Antonio

Robert P. Wilder, M.D., F.A.C.S.M.
Director, Sports Rehabilitation Services, Department of Physical Medicine and Rehabilitation, The Tom Landry Sports Medicine and Research Center, Baylor University Medical Center, Dallas

Preface

The aquatic environment has provided therapeutic benefits throughout the millennia. Most early aquatic venues were derivatives of natural locations: mineral pools, ocean waters, streams, and springs. The development of specific aquatic rehabilitation techniques arose largely from the evolution of earlier techniques translated into new aquatic environments. Techniques were modified to suit mineral spring temperatures; variations in saline or mineral content, which altered buoyancy and required adaptations in treatment methods; and advances in science and materials, which allowed and suggested a broader range of treatment options. This evolutionary trend has continued to the present.

Health care became more formally centered within the hospital environment during the early part of this century, especially in North America; a decreasing reliance was placed on the spa as a health care option. Although some hospitals had therapeutic pools and most had hydrotherapy departments with Hubbard tanks and whirlpool baths, treatment in the aquatic environment was a peripheral part of health care. The use of aquatic rehabilitation techniques did not grow during this time and, often, the advantages of water as a treatment medium were forgotten or ignored in the press of time and energy within the health care system.

As health care reimbursement has become increasingly controlled by the third-party payment system, treatment methods such as aquatic rehabilitation are often neglected because other, more economically productive, though sometimes less effective, techniques can be used. Aquatic therapy is placed at a disadvantage because many clinical effects are achieved during a treatment session, but current billing systems force the practitioner to pick only one effect per session or to bundle the charge. For example, during a typical aquatic treatment session with a patient with a hip fracture, the patient is exposed to hydrostatic pressure, which drives out edema around the fracture site and in the distal limb while increasing circulation to the fracture site. At the same time, the patient is moving the limb through an increasing range of motion, while exerting muscle force to strengthen the muscles across the hip joint and preserve strength elsewhere. The same patient initiates walking with the forces of gravity reduced by water buoyancy while working on gait training and balance activities. But the therapist cannot bill for each beneficial effect; instead he or she must choose an arbitrary "most important" effect, or bundle the treatment charge under "pool therapy." A single session in the pool might achieve many treatment benefits, in a shorter time and at lower cost than billing for many benefits individually. In the fee-for-service health care system, it is much more profitable to pick the latter course. Thus, there has also been an economic force behind the decline in aquatic therapeutics. This decline has been aggravated by the decrease in curriculum time devoted to the techniques and rationale of aquatic rehabilitation in both medical and physical therapy education.

During the second half of this century, fewer hospitals have included pools as a part of their construction because of expense and maintenance. Physical therapy departments have devoted less space to hydrotherapy departments because of the diminishing role hydrotherapy has had in contemporary health care. Rehabilitation hospitals usually include pools and often use these pools for group activities and sometimes for recreational purposes for rehabilitation patients, but there is little crossover between the community pool and the therapeutic pool and virtually no crossover between the other aquatic rehabilitation venues in use in hospitals and the community.

As a consequence, a communication gap has developed among these various facilities and among the personnel responsible for the care of the public in each. Physical therapists have tended to practice in isolation, therapeutic recreation personnel have developed their own programs, organizations such as the Red Cross have created programs on their own, and overall there has been minimal interaction with the health care system. As a result, a babel of systems, techniques, and turf barriers has evolved.

Better coordination is required to optimize the potential of aquatic therapy. The aquatic environment has a broad margin of therapeutic safety and can be used in the management of a wide range of issues, from the formal medical management of specific diseases to the recreational use by multigenerational populations. The continuum of care from acute disease management to general health and well-being can be aided by the aquatic environment. The current gaps in understanding of the physiologic benefits of water, treatment techniques, and methods to mesh the health care system with the community do not serve the public.

Aquatic facilities are expensive to build and maintain. Many pool facilities are underutilized, especially during daytime hours. Rehabilitation may safely and economically occur in these community facilities, but members of the health care system often overlook their availability and utility. At the same time, current health care costs are widely viewed as too high. Scarcely an issue of the newspaper is published without a reference to changes in the health care system to decrease costs. Thus, perhaps the logical direction of aquatic therapy is to narrow the physical and communication gaps between the health care system and the community pool, to extend the hospital into the community, and vice versa.

Another important element is at play in the aquatic therapy environment. Even the most casual visitor to the rehabilitation pool will notice an important difference from almost any other treatment venue: the sound of laughter. There is something within the human soul that is liberated upon immersion. Patients with acute illnesses, those with severely disabling conditions, and children in pain can all be seen smiling and relaxed in the pool. Those familiar with Ron Howard's movie "Cocoon" will remember the seniors at play in the pool, suddenly transformed from their geriatric status into the mental frame of rowdy children. There is no medical term for this phenomenon, but only the most callous health care provider would deny its value in the therapeutic process.

In conceiving this book, the authors have responded to the requests of a broad range of aquatic professionals who felt there was a need to summarize the effects of the aquatic environment on human physiology, to bring forward new advances in treatment methodologies, and to describe the current state of the aquatic rehabilitation art. In so doing, we have attempted to detail the scientific underpinnings that are the foundation of all aquatic therapies and build these foundations into the treatment rationales in current use. We hope that we have succeeded in creating a reference that will facilitate the transfer of knowledge of the great number of biological processes affected by the aquatic environment. We also hope to enable aquatic practitioners to develop their own methods and techniques built on this scientific understanding, as well as on the heads and shoulders of the careful and visionary treatment innovators who went before.

The aquatic environment has tremendous utility in these times of health care containment: to transfer medical treatment efficiently into the community setting, to build fitness and conditioning as a lifestyle, and to rebuild the community pool into a health and wellness center integrated with the health care system would be a great service to the population. This is not a revolutionary idea: One only has to examine the design of the most advanced ancient Roman baths to realize that society has come this way before. Thus, we have begun to close the circle historically, adding a great deal of science and technology along the way to better understand the processes and reasons for aquatic therapy. Let us all work together toward this closure.

B.E.B.
A.J.C.

Acknowledgments

A great number of individuals have facilitated the process of writing this book. My parents were perhaps the central people in the development of my interest in aquatic therapy. It was they who followed the aquatic and physical therapy recommendations of the Sister Kenny Hospital staff in assisting my recovery from poliomyelitis as a child in Minneapolis, and I shall remain grateful for life. My adult learning about aquatic rehabilitation has been fostered by many individuals. Drs. Luis de-Lerma, Herman Flax, Jens Henrickson, Chester Wong, and Robert Christopher were all instrumental in the early days of the American Society of Medical Hydrology, supporting Dr. Sidney Licht in keeping the organizational flames alive through the years of bridging the gap between the therapy world and formal medicine, while linking to the established strong traditions of the International Society of Medical Hydrology. Their support of the organization and assistance during my years as president of the organization have been tremendously helpful.

My interest in aquatic therapy was greatly expanded by many people during my years in Eugene, Oregon. Juliana Larson was the engine and fuel behind the development of the Eugene aquatic rehabilitative community, cheerleading, guiding, demonstrating by example and knowledge the pathways to healing. Juliana's "mermaidens," her circle of aquatic gurus from across the nation, who tolerated my ignorant questions and guided the linkages back to medicine, were immensely helpful and continue to be so today. Many are represented within these covers. Richard Brown, Ph.D., was active during the early years of SciEx, Inc. and was responsible for the development of many of the track and field aquatic rehabilitative programs that SciEx put together. My physician partners in Rehabilitation Medicine Associates, particularly Martha MacRitchie, Bryan Andresen, and Rod Cox, were supportive of the aquatic mission and tolerant of the time and energy that was diverted to my hydrorehabilitation activities. Pam Perkins and Shelly Postle provided critical organizational counsel and advice to SciEx throughout its history.

My wife Carol, daughter Adrianne, and son Derek have paid heavily for my efforts in these areas, giving up time that could have been spent with them, and missing paternal involvement in activities that should have had a father's representation. Their love and forgiveness have been critical. Lastly, I would like to thank my coauthor Andy Cole, who has been a major source of energy, enthusiasm, and creativity through many years of collaboration. Without Andy, this book and our many other joint efforts in the field might not have happened.

B.E.B.

I will always be grateful to my Chairman, John Downey, M.D., D.Phil. (Oxon), F.R.C.P.(C), for introducing me to the benefits of aquatic rehabilitation and to Marilou Moschetti, P.T.; Richard Eagleston, A.T.C., P.T.; and Steven Stratton, Ph.D., P.T., A.T.C., for expanding my aquatic horizons. I am deeply appreciative for the support of Robert Christopher, M.D.; Luis deLerma, M.D.; Herman Flax, M.D.; and Jans Henrickson, M.D. I am also indebted to my colleague Sandra Pinkerton, Ph.D., for helping me become a better writer and to Bruce Becker, M.D., for his support and inspiration during our many collaborative efforts.

Finally, thanks to Avalon, Merlin, and Morgane for the long hours spent quietly keeping me company on top of my computer.

A.J.C.

1

Aquatic Rehabilitation:
An Historical Perspective

Jonathan Paul De Vierville

A NEW BRANCH ON AN OLD TREE

Aquatic rehabilitation is a new name for a treatment method with ancient roots. Over the centuries, health care practitioners have used various terms for the therapeutic and rehabilitative benefits conferred by water. *Aquatic rehabilitation* is a late-twentieth century term that describes a scientific theory, medical rationale, and a set of clinical procedures using water immersion for the restoration of physical mobility and physiologic activity, and, at times, for effecting psychological transformation.

As a recently developed medical treatment modality, aquatic rehabilitation has a relatively brief history. When linked with the lengthy history of healing waters, thermal baths, health resort medicine, and spa therapies, however, aquatic rehabilitation serves as a contemporary affirmation of the classic medical traditions that used healing water pools. In this sense, contemporary aquatic rehabilitation can trace its origins from the first civilizations.

ORIGINS OF AQUATIC THERAPY

Humans, especially the sick and suffering, have long resorted to springs, baths, and pools for their soothing and healing properties. Taking the waters, soaking in baths and pools, and resting at places called spas played an important social and spiritual role in the river valley civilizations of Mesopotamia, Egypt, India, and China. Ritual bathing pools were widely used for individual, religious, and social renewal and healing.\Healing water rituals also appeared in ancient Greek, Hebrew, Roman, Christian, and Islamic cultures. Ancient civilizations used the waters for cleaning the earthly body of disease and cleansing the spiritual body of sin. These cultures taught that clean bodies and pure souls facilitated seasonal as well as eternal renewal, which in turn ensured cultural regeneration.

Swiss cultural historian Sigfried Giedion made the following observation:

> The bath and its purposes have held different meanings for different ages. The manner in which a civilization integrates bathing within its life, as well as the type of bathing it prefers, yields searching insight into the inner nature of the period. . . . The role that bathing plays

within a culture reveals the culture's attitude toward human relaxation. It is a measure of how far individual well-being is regarded as an indispensable part of community life [1].

Giedion explains the bath and its role in two types of regenerative processes: individual and social. Individual bathing is a private hygienic act of body care known as an *ablution*. The other type of regenerative process is social bathing, a receptive, relaxed, and restorative activity that enhances wellness for the whole being and embodies the "broad ideal [of] total regeneration" [1].

THE SPA CONCEPT

Much of the current field of aquatic rehabilitation has its roots in the European and early American spa world. Etymologically, *spa* is traced from the Latin verb *spargere*, to pour forth. Roman legions built their camps at hot springs, where healing waters "poured forth." The modern word *spa* found its way into the English language through the old Walloon word *espa*, which referred to a fountain. From *espa* the English derived *spaw*. In 1326, at a little village located in the Ardennes range, the name *Spa* was used to identify some hot mineral springs discovered to possess therapeutic and medicinal values. Shortly thereafter, pools were built at Spa, Belgium. Two-hundred and twenty-five years later, William Slingsby discovered the sulfur springs of Tewhit near Harrogate, England and compared these natural sulfur mineral fountains to those at Spa, Belgium.

In the 1950s, Dr. Sidney Licht, a founding member of the American Society of Medical Hydrology and Climatology, defined a spa as a "place where mineral containing waters flow from the ground naturally, or to which [they are] pumped or conducted, and [are] there used for therapeutic purposes" [2]. Similarly, Dr. Walter S. McClellan, the first medical director of the Saratoga Spa in Saratoga Springs, New York, considered a spa "a place or location where nature has provided natural healing agents such as mineral waters or peloids, at which provisions have been made in physical plant and equipment for the administration of treatments which utilize[s] these agents, and where the program is carried out under medical control" [3]. Thus, the historical definition of the spa recognizes an important social institution that provides a time and place for activities, leisure, relaxation, healing, and renewal. The spa concept spawned development of the foundations of contemporary aquatic rehabilitation.

GREEK, ROMAN, AND MEDIEVAL SPA CULTURES

Social bathing as a component of individual and cultural recreation was an important part of the cultures of the ancient Greeks and Romans. The Greeks believed in the relationship between the gymnastic invigoration of the body and the academic stimulation of the mind (Figures 1-1 and 1-2). The buildings at Delphi (334 BC) included the gymnasium, xystos (track), and palaestra with its loutron (cold water washroom), and ephebeum. The ephebeum, the large main room, was used for educational and social functions. Similar to Delphi, the Sanctuary of Zeus at Olympia shows the large gymnasium in close proximity to the palaestra, with its loutron. Other bathing arrangements of the era resembled those at the Greek colony (310–280 BC) of Gela (Sicily), where individual tubs are set in a line and in a circle [4]. Parallel to current practice, bathing followed exercise, and was believed to have therapeutic value.

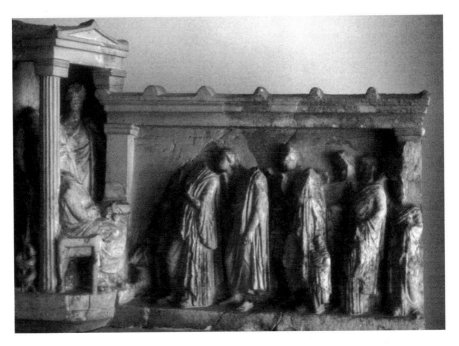

Figure 1-1. Ancient (circa 340 BC) bas relief from the Sanctuary of Aesculapius at Epidaurus, Greece.

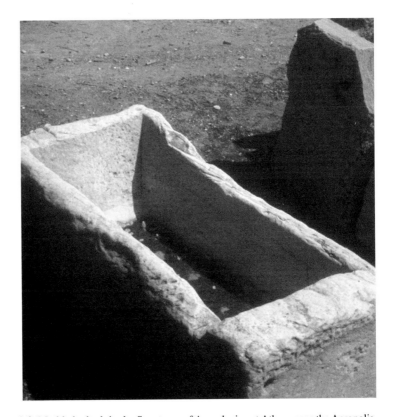

Figure 1-2. Marble bathtub in the Sanctuary of Aesculapius at Athens near the Acropolis.

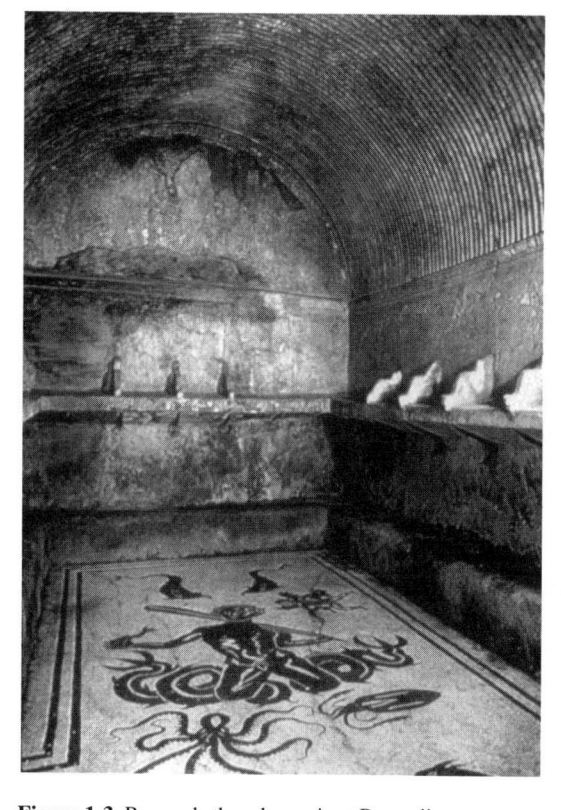

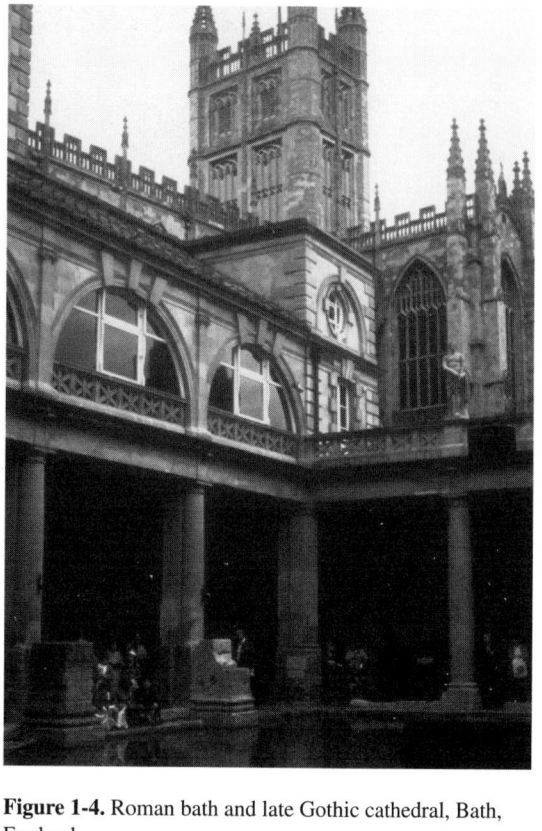

Figure 1-3. Roman bath and mosaic at Pompeii.

Figure 1-4. Roman bath and late Gothic cathedral, Bath, England.

Whereas the Greeks considered bathing an added function to the gymnasium, the Romans considered bathing a central social function to accompany activities that might include exercise in a gymnasium. Roman culture elevated bathing practices to a more practical, formal, educational, social, and technically refined level (Figure 1-3). Roman *thermae*, including hot-air baths, frigid pools, and relaxation areas, functioned as an important social and civil institution and enabled usage that was believed to be medically beneficial. The physician Galen had his office in the baths of Hadrian.

The Roman thermae contained multiple rooms and pools with varied temperatures and an ambulacrum with space for libraries, lecture rooms, art and sculpture galleries, multipurpose meeting and ceremonial halls, shaded parks and promenades, small theaters, indoor athletic halls, and, occasionally, sports stadiums. Behind the scenes were the furnaces and service areas for wood, food, and laundry. The first public baths in Rome, and possibly the first in the series of imperial thermae, are believed to be the Baths of Agrippa, built in 25 BC [4].

Following the decline of the western Roman Empire, Byzantium carried on the thermae traditions in the East. Islamic culture later replaced the active games and athletics with scrubs and massages, which became a central part of the traditional Turkish bath. Russian culture combined hot vapor baths with cold plunges. The Russian steam bath may be one of the oldest forms of social bathing for physical, spiritual, and cultural regeneration.

In Europe during the Middle Ages, grand healing pools were built around thermal springs in Aachen, Poretta, Baden-Baden, Bath (Figure 1-4), and Spa, Belgium. As

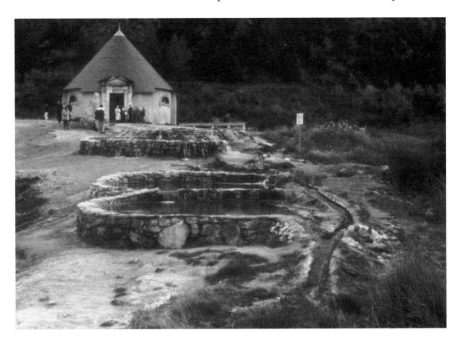

Figure 1-5. Mountain baths from the Middle Ages, France.

early as 740 AD in Switzerland, the Benedictine Abbey of Pfäfers served as the spiritual and cultural center of Switzerland. Here the mountain monks operated the baths of Pfäfers, where during the Renaissance the new humanists came to meet and talk. In 1535, Theophrastus of Hohenheim, better known as Paracelsus, practiced his healing arts at Bad Pfäfers. By the nineteenth century, Bad Ragaz (Switzerland) had developed into a major health resort spa, where today the aquatic rehabilitation procedure known as the Bad Ragaz ring method is taught and practiced. Similar aquatic histories and traditions are found at other European spas, including Aix-les-Bains, Evian-les-Bains, Vichy, Baden-Baden, Motecatini Terme, Albano, San Pellegrino, Karlsbad, Marienbad, and Franzbad (Figure 1-5). These sites have served European medicine for centuries, and even today many are part of standard traditional health care practice.

GROWTH OF AQUATIC THERAPY IN AMERICA

The European history of aquatic traditions is lengthy, as is America's. New World natives practiced similar hot air and cold plunge baths in the sweat lodge, which served both medical and religious purposes. Since Ponce de Leon's search and de Soto's trek through the New World forests, America's healing waters have been discovered, lost, and rediscovered with each generation. In the 1600s, the English, Dutch, and French colonists built their stone huts and wooden tubs near wilderness healing springs frequented by Indians. During the 1700s, natural philosophers such as Drs. John de Normandie and Benjamin Rush traveled to the colonial mineral springs and thermal pools to analyze the waters for their chemical and medicinal virtues. In Virginia, Thomas

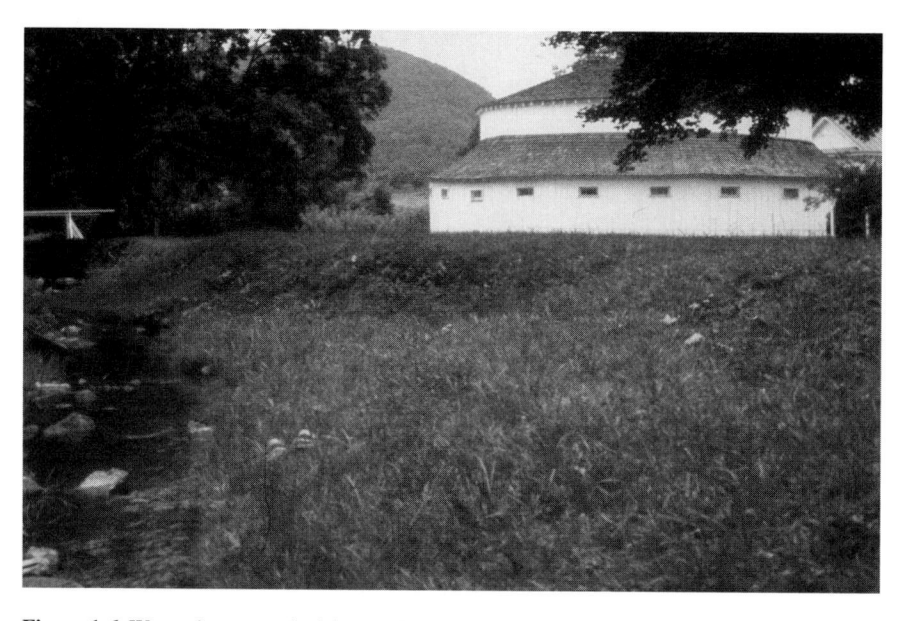

Figure 1-6. Women's octagon bath house, Warm Springs, Virginia.

Jefferson rode his horse to the distant Warm Springs Valley and made notes on the healing mineral springs and pools (Figure 1-6). Jefferson used Palladio's ancient Roman drawings to design the Sweet Springs spa in West Virginia.

In the decades before the Civil War, major health reforms swept the nation, and numerous hydropathic establishments, institutes, and medical colleges were built for the practice of the *water cure* (cold water bathing). Health reformers, including Dr. and Mrs. Shew, Dr. Russell Trall, Dr. Nichols, and Mary Gove-Nichols wrote lengthy books on bathing practices, and spa doctors traveled to distant frontier springs. Others, such as Dr. Thomas Goode of the Homestead and Dr. John Jennings Moorman of the Greenbrier, developed notable medical reputations for their aquatic treatments (Figure 1-7). Western pioneers, such as Hiram Abiff Whittington at Hot Springs, Arkansas, constructed large thermal pools for traveling invalids.

During the era of Reconstruction, Dr. George G. Walton analyzed many newly discovered frontier springs and constructed an elaborate scientific classification system of the springs based on geography, climatology, mineralogy, chemistry, and geology. In 1880, the American Medical Association (AMA) Committee on Sanitaria and Springs published its first national report on sanitaria. The AMA committee classified the nation's 646 known springs and mineral water pools. Several years later, Dr. Albert Charles Peale classified 2,822 active therapeutic springs. By 1896, 19 spa doctors using the healing waters and thermal pools at Hot Springs, Arkansas, had published their medical theories and cases in the *Hot Springs Medical Journal*.

AMERICAN SPAS IN THE TWENTIETH CENTURY

At the turn of the century, medical men like Simon Baruch, John Harvey Kellogg, and Guy Hinsdale regularly conducted clinical hydrotherapeutic experiments and prescribed what were termed *balneotherapeutics*. They also recommended clima-

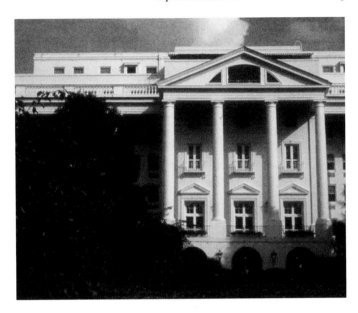

Figure 1-7. The Greenbrier at White Sulphur Springs, West Virginia.

totherapeutics and sent their patients to mountain springs where clean air and sunshine provided healthy environments. Baruch established the American medical standards for hydrotherapy in his *Principles and Practice of Hydrotherapy* (Figure 1-8). Kellogg, who directed the Battle Creek Sanitarium in Michigan, published an enormous volume on hydrotherapy, which included his scientific theories and practices of hydrotherapy based on a systematic but iconoclastic and controversial physiologic system for internal and external aquatic treatments. After World War I, Dr. H.H. Roberts published an examination of the therapeutic value of America's health resorts and spas for rehabilitation [5]. In 1920, Simon Baruch published his last book, *An Epitome of Hydrotherapy*. An international journal, the *Archives of Medical Hydrology* began publication in 1922 (Figure 1-9).

Although most spa doctors wrote about and prescribed the internal and external curative benefits of water, baths, and pools, they usually placed limited emphasis on water exercise. Most bathing activities in America were passive. As early as 1911, however, Dr. Charles LeRoy Lowman was using therapeutic tubs to treat patients with cerebral palsy and spastic conditions. Lowman, who founded the Orthopaedic Hospital in Los Angeles in 1913 (now Rancho Los Amigos), visited the Spaulding School for Crippled Children in Chicago, where he observed paralyzed patients exercising in a wooden tank. On his return to California, he transformed the hospital's lily pond into two therapeutic pools. One fresh-water pool was used for therapy with paralyzed and poliomyelitis patients; the other pool was filled with saline water and used to treat patients with infectious diseases. He also made a motion picture showing the various types of cases treated with pool therapy [6]. At Warm Springs, Georgia, LeRoy Hubbard developed his famous tank, and, in 1924, Warm Springs received its most famous aquatic patient, Franklin D. Roosevelt. Still a private citizen, Roosevelt traveled to Georgia, where he exercised his withered legs. A decade later, newsreels showed the crippled President Roosevelt performing therapeutic water exercises, which encouraged the medical acceptance of aquatic rehabilitation.

Before the Great Depression, America's spas experienced rapid expansion. When the stock market crashed, however, spas did not immediately feel the impact. In fact, the publicly owned spas, such as Saratoga Springs and Hot Springs, Arkansas, benefited from the Depression: More people visited spas for therapeutic reasons, and the wealthy, who could no longer afford travel to Europe, chose American pools [7]. At the Homestead, Drs. Frank Hopkins and Melius Jarman described the expanded Hot Springs Spa as a place in America where a professional medical staff administered the ancient "Aesculapian art" [8].

At Saratoga, financier Bernard M. Baruch, Roosevelt's friend and the son of Simon Baruch, headed a special commission. The Baruch Commission was formed with the assistance of the New York Academy of Medicine and comprised a geologist from Columbia University, a committee of five physicians, and Dr. Franz Groedel, a notable European balneologist. Groedel, later a founder and president of the American College of Cardiology [9], was then a professor at the State University, Frankfurt-am-Main, and director of the Kerckhoff Institute at Bad Nauheim. The Commission planned a scientific American spa [10], studied spa design, natural treatments, and efficient operations based on sound medical and scientific care for

SPA DESIGN, RESEARCH, AND THE DEPRESSION YEARS

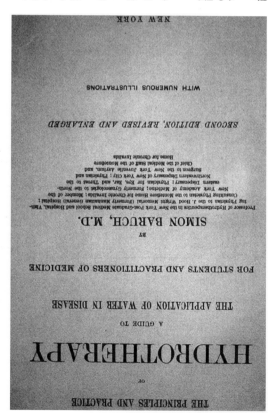

Figure 1-8. Title page for Dr. Simon Baruch's book *Principles and Practice of Hydrotherapy.*

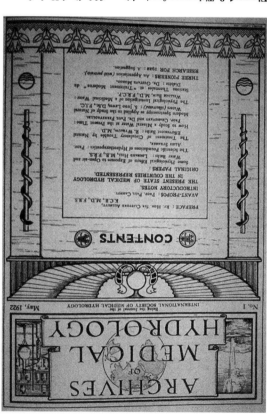

Figure 1-9. Title page for *Archives of Medical Hydrology.*

chronically ill patients, especially those suffering from cardiac, vascular, and circulatory ailments [11]. Groedel's work at Saratoga and subsequent scientific lectures provided a major medical contribution to American health resort medicine, spa therapy, and aquatic rehabilitation [12]. The Commission selected McClellan as medical spa director [10]. His first task at Saratoga Spa was to design a new spa research laboratory, for which he recruited help from Dr. W.E. Fitch, author of the 1927 comprehensive volume, *Mineral Waters of the United States and American Spas*. Fitch was the medical director at French Lick Springs Hotel and Spa in Indiana, which was staffed and equipped with the best available hydrotherapeutic department. (It was at French Lick Spa during the 1931 summer National Governors Convention that Governor Franklin Roosevelt initially gathered support for his presidential bid.)

Also in 1931, Fitch, McClellan, and several others, scientific directors, general managers, and others met at French Lick Spa with the purpose of organizing "an association which would be of mutual benefit to everyone interested in the advancement of Medical Hydrology in this country" [13]. Participants reviewed a half-century of American spa programs. Their discussion anticipated spa therapy and aquatic rehabilitation for the following 50 years [13]. Shortly thereafter, Groedel came to New York to help design Saratoga's Spa.

During the Depression years, investigators researched the physical, psychiatric, thermal, mechanical, chemical, mineral, electrical, and radioactive qualities of the American spa waters, and medical organizations held special meetings and conducted spa tours. A wealth of information, research, and articles on health resort medicine, spa therapy, and pool treatments appeared in the professional journals of that time. At Northwestern University Medical School in Chicago, Dr. John S. Coulter, the first full-time academic physician in physical medicine, presented lectures on physical therapy, which he placed within the history of spa medicine [14]. In Boston, Dr. Rebekah Wright, a psychiatrist employed by the Massachusetts Department of Mental Diseases, researched the use of water for its psychotherapeutic effects. In her book, *Hydrotherapy in Psychiatric Hospitals*, Wright described 32 aquatically based procedures used to achieve sedative, stimulating, anodyne, hypnotic, eliminative, and antipyretic effects on the body [15]. In 1933, America's healing waters were officially recognized with the establishment of the Simon Baruch Research Institute of Balneology at Saratoga Springs Spa and the printing of a series of scientific bulletins. At Hot Springs National Park in Arkansas, another group of spa doctors, including Louis G. Martin [16], Euclid Smith [17], George B. Fletcher [18], and Nelda King [19], physical therapist at the Maurice Baths, researched and practiced pool therapy and underwater physiotherapy. In 1936, Roosevelt traveled by special presidential train to Hot Springs, where he visited the Army and Navy Hospital and Bath House Row. The same year, Dr. Albert W. Wallace described America's health resort spas and their full medical potential in the *Journal of the American Medical Association* (*JAMA*) [20]. He listed 10 universal spa features.

1. Proper use of mineral springs and climates
2. Competent medical supervision
3. Proper dietary regimen
4. Systematic rest
5. Regulated exercise
6. Proper knowledge of the patient's reserve and limits

7. Spa therapies, including physical, electric, heliotherapeutic, and hydrotherapeutic procedures administered by competent attendants
8. Planning and regulation of the patient's day
9. Elevation of the morale
10. Development of a proper perspective (patient's and doctor's) toward the disease from which the patient suffers

Spa medicine at that time used large pools and tanks. In the basement pool of the
Maurice Bath House at Hot Springs, Arkansas, a warm swimming pool was installed
in the 1930s for underwater physical therapy exercises and pool therapy treatments
with chronic arthritic patients [17]. By 1937, Lowman published *Technique of
Underwater Gymnastics: A Study in Practical Application*, in which he detailed pool
therapy methods of specific underwater exercises that "carefully regulated dosage,
character, frequency, and duration for remedying bodily deformities and restoring
muscle function" [6]. This was one of the earliest American publications on what
has evolved into aquatic rehabilitation, and it was a landmark effort to quantify the
aquatic regimen.

At the Fifteenth Congress of Physical Therapy in 1936, Groedel [21], McClellan
[22], and Behrend [23] presented papers on spa medicine research. As a result of the
Sixteenth Congress, a three-page editorial on American health resorts appeared in
the *Archives of Physical Therapy, X-Ray and Radium*, and a Committee on Spas
and Health Resorts in the United States was formed [24]. The committee's first action established a formal outline for a national survey (WS McClellan, personal
communication, 1936). Physicians subsequently toured spas at French Lick, Battle
Creek, and Mount Clemens in Michigan, and Glens Springs, Richfield Springs,
Sharon Springs, and Saratoga Springs in New York. In 1937, a resolution was
drafted calling for the AMA to establish a council on spas and health resorts [25].
Dr. Bernard Fantus convinced Morris Fishbein, editor of *JAMA*, to publish a special
article requesting that the AMA "study the vital importance of active medical programs for spas and health resorts" [26]. The following year, a second spa tour group
visited Bedford Springs, Pennsylvania, the Homestead, the Greenbrier, and French
Lick Spa, ending its tour at the Seventeenth Congress in Chicago, where the Committee on Spas and Health Resorts presented a full report [27,28]. The AMA understood the therapeutic significance and growing interest in spas and appointed its
own committee, but the trustees did not like the historical reputation of America's
spas and insisted that the only suitable term was *health resort*, not *spa*. *JAMA* published numerous articles affirming the value of "health resort" therapy for "chronic
disabling conditions, including those affecting the heart and circulation, rheumatic
disorders, ailments of the stomach, intestinal tract, gallbladder and liver, nervous
conditions, certain disorders of the skin and some metabolic diseases" [28]. Even
Medical Economics published an article on the medical and economic implications
of spa medicine [29].

WAR, PHYSICAL MEDICINE, AND SPA
REHABILITATION CENTERS

The Depression and later the medical consequences of the second World War benefited American spas. In 1941, there were a total of 8,826 mineral springs at 2,717 different locations with 321 spas and health resort facilities [30], but there were no

major national organization, certification, or accrediting bodies. Medicine was changing, with increased specialization, and was generally organized along organ systems. Although Drs. Coulter and Frank H. Krusen led the organization of the American Academy of Physical Medicine in 1938, no specialty included the multi-disciplinary practice of health resort medicine, spa therapy, and aquatic rehabilitation as a central theme. Even though the AMA did define certain minimum health resort standards based on established scientific procedure, references in the medical litera-ture, especially to spa therapy and natural therapeutic agents and resources, were generally ignored.

Dr. Henry Sigerist, a leading medical historian of that time and founder of the *Bulletin of the History of Medicine*, tried to keep the waters flowing by writing about the history of American spas [31]. But 1941 was a time for war, not for spa organiz-ing or teaching. The war forced major changes on America's spas and their treat-ment methods. The Army, the Navy, and the Veterans Administration commandeered some of the best spas and turned them into military hospitals for physical therapy and rehabilitation programs [32]. Despite the war, *JAMA* published a special series of 18 articles on health resort therapy between October 1943 and May 1947.

Following the war, a new Commission on Physical Medicine was established and chaired by Krusen. A member of the AMA Health Resort Committee and a rig-orous scientist, Krusen was skeptical about health resort medicine and spa therapy, although he was a firm believer in the therapeutic value of medical hydrology as a part of a grander concept. He promoted physical medicine and rehabilitation, a sub-ject he taught at the Mayo Clinic. Krusen, the first to use the term *physiatrist*, played a key role in the development of postwar physical medicine and rehabilita-tion, especially as a newly developed medical specialty.

The Commission on Physical Medicine Subcommittee for Medical Hydrology and Health Resorts reported on the future of spa health resorts as rehabilitation cen-ters [33]. The report assessed the needs for basic research, teaching, clinical prac-tice, and rehabilitation in the field of hydrotherapy as related to physiologic changes that occurred in the circulation, respiration, metabolism, and body chemistry during water treatments. Several American spas offered medically supervised regimens, and a few orthopedic and mental hospitals practiced hydrotherapy, but scientific research was sparse. The military hospitals at Hot Springs, Arkansas; Glenwood Springs, Colorado; and Saratoga Springs, New York, operated institutional spa reha-bilitation centers. The report recommended the establishment of spa rehabilitation centers throughout the country at health resorts. Besides treating war veterans, spa rehabilitation centers also treated patients injured in industrial jobs, patients suffer-ing from chronic degenerative diseases, and patients in post-hospital convalescence. Unfortunately, the Committee on Physical Medicine did not include these recom-mendations in its final report. The interest and organizational support for health re-sort medicine, spa therapy, and aquatic rehabilitation had diminished significantly by the war's end.

POSTWAR POOLS AND MEDICAL HYDROLOGY

Postwar American culture focused on the powers of science and technology, and rel-atively few physicians remembered how earlier civilized cultures used and revered the regenerative powers of healing waters. During the early 1950s, as poliomyelitis affected nearly 58,000 Americans annually, the National Foundation for Infantile

Paralysis supported the corrective swimming pools and hydrogymnastics of Lowman and the therapeutic use of pools and tanks for the treatment of poliomyelitis. But with the development of the Salk vaccine and the subsequent demise of poliomyelitis in the later 1950s, the medical perception of need for complex aquatic therapy regimens waned, and pools became far less important to hospital practice. Pools went into disrepair, and therapists began to lose interest in and understanding of the old techniques. The advances made immediately before and during the war years, followed by the increased understanding gains during the polio era, began to fade.

By 1962, however, Drs. Licht, Herman Flax, Sigmund Foster, William Erdman, Lucille Eising, J. Wayne McFarland, Jens Henriksen, and Richard Gubner recognized the need for torchbearers to keep medical hydrology knowledge alive. They organized the American Society of Medical Hydrology and Climatology (ASMH) as the North American affiliate for the International Society of Medical Hydrology and Climatology (ISMH). Since 1921, the ISMH, as the World Congress for Health Resort Medicine and Spa Therapy, has been meeting every 4 years around the world. ISMH has a long-established international history and publishes statutes and standards for health resort medicine and spa therapy. The Thirty-Second World Congress of ISMH (1994) was held in Bad Wörishofen, Germany, the historical spa town of Father Sebastian Kneipp, one of the legendary figures in modern medical hydrology (Figure 1-10).

The late 1960s and early 1970s were a golden time in American basic science research. Research funds were plentiful as we attempted to move into space. During this period of Space Age research, as Dr. Bruce Becker points out, scientists "began to study the effects of weightlessness through research in water, the only environment that could approximate the effects of space flight" [34].

In 1969, Neil Armstrong first walked on the moon. In the same year, several other historic events occurred relating to aquatic environments, therapies, and rehabilitation. In January, the first issue of the *Medical Hydrology Quarterly* appeared under the editorship of Henriksen. This issue contained a report on Dr. V.R. Ott's lecture on spa cardiac rehabilitation to the 1968 ASMH annual meeting, in which he made the following observation:

> The need for spa courses today seems as vital as in those olden times when spa vacations were stipulated in marriage contracts of wealthy citizens and when people believed that bathing in mineral wells was diving into a miracle fountain and becoming rejuvenated by decades. Present medicine should not neglect the possibilities of adapting an age-old principle to modern science and to the philosophy of rehabilitation [35].

What was written 3 decades ago holds true today and for future research, development, education, and practice of comprehensive aquatic therapies and rehabilitation.

HEALTH SPAS AND AQUATICS ORGANIZE

In 1991, the International Spa and Fitness Association organized its first international conference and trade exposition, dubbed "The Ultimate Workout." In attendance were 150 delegates from 20 states and 10 countries, including spa owners, managers, marketing and public relations directors, nutritionists, chefs, massage therapists, estheticians, trainers, consultants, travel agents, government officials, airlines, and equipment and supply vendors. But conspicuously absent

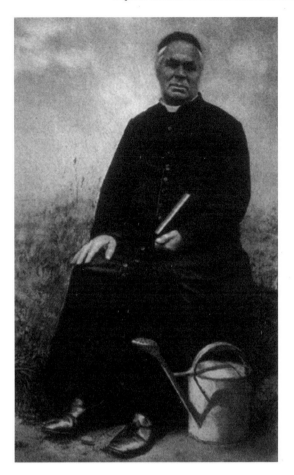

Figure 1-10. Father Sebastian Kneipp.

from this group was any significant representation from the medical establishment. The scientific rationalization of the 1950s, 1960s, and 1970s had engineered a divorce between the mind and the body, with medicine assuming responsibility for the body.

In 1989, Bernard Burt published a list of health resorts in the first edition of *Fodor's Health and Fitness Vacations* [36]. Taking a vacation for health reasons was not a new concept, nor was a list of resorts and spas, telling travelers where they could find the needed health resources. What was new and important about Burt's guide was its listing of health resort and spa resources, not only by region but also by the types of fitness programs and health spa treatments. The book lists 12 categories of programs, including luxury pampering, life enhancement, weight management, nutrition and diet, stress control, holistic health, spiritual awareness, preventive medicine, "taking the waters," sports conditioning, youth camps for weight loss, and nonprogram resort facilities. Although it is useful for health seekers looking for wellness and fitness, the book contained little information on affiliation with formal medicine. The public had responded to medicine's disregard for spa medicine by viewing established medicine as irrelevant to the New Age concept of wellness.

But the increasing public interest combined with the neglect of formal training in the principles of aquatic rehabilitation began to create a hunger in professionals working in the area. Interest grew within the American Physical Therapy Association (APTA). The Aquatic Exercise Association (AEA) was established in the mid-1980s to provide professional development, services, and products related to aquatic fitness and aquatic therapy industries for allied health care professionals, including physical and occupational therapists, kinesiotherapists, recreational and aquatic therapists, and aerobics instructors. AEA publishes The AKWA Letter and offers workshops and certification programs for aquatic instructors and pool specialists. A related organization, the Aquatic Therapy and Rehabilitation Institute (ATRI) has labored to develop multidisciplinary standards for aquatic therapy. It is important to note the differentiation between AEA's focus on aquatic exercise and ATRI's focus on aquatic therapy. Together, the AEA and ATRI host an Annual Aquatic Symposium with many workshops conducted in aquatic environments, as well as formal classroom instruction. Organizations such as these may play an important role in the future development and expansion of American comprehensive aquatic rehabilitation. Paralleling the growth of these organizations has been the development of a large special interest section within the APTA, led by several of the contributors to this book.

AN AQUATIC RENAISSANCE

Aquatics as applied to health and rehabilitation is experiencing a renaissance. Many professional groups and organizations claim an interest in America's healing waters. Besides those already mentioned, this list includes the American Academy of Physical Medicine and Rehabilitation, with its own special interest aquatic rehabilitation group, the American Congress of Physical Medicine and Rehabilitation, the Council for National Cooperation in Aquatics, the National Museum and Educational Center for Allied Healthcare Professionals, the American Kinesiotherapy Association, National Spa and Pool Institute, and the American Red Cross Water Safety Instructor Certification.

This renaissance has parallels in most areas of scientific interest. A waxing of enthusiasm is followed by development of a field, which is, in turn, followed by waning interest and consolidation of some of the gains achieved, with loss of some others. The current rebirth of aquatic therapy signals a new milestone along a road that began in ancient times with Aesculapius and the thermae of Rome and continued through Byzantium, Russia, and Europe, leading to modern corporate American medicine. The belief in the therapeutic effects of water continue today. The cultural perceptions, ideas, and theories are reflected in the value placed on the aquatic environment. Contemporary aquatic rehabilitation is rediscovering and redefining the aquatic traditions established earlier in this century by medical hydrology, health resort medicine, and spa therapy.

American health care practitioners are looking again at the aquatic environment as a safe, effective, and inexpensive way of using water to preserve health and treat disease. In this way our civilization will reconnect to the ancient aquatic traditions of healing, rejuvenation, and repair.

REFERENCES

1. Giedion S. Part VII: The Mechanization of the Bath. In S Giedion (ed), Mechanization Takes Command, A Contribution to Anonymous History. Oxford, England: Oxford University Press, 1948;628.
2. Licht S (ed). Medical Hydrology. The Physical Medicine Library, Vol 7. Baltimore: Waverly, 1963;437.
3. McClellan WS. Spa therapy. Interne 1946;(Oct):674.
4. Yegül F. Baths and Bathing in Classical Antiquity. Cambridge, MA: MIT Press, 1992;9, 49, 490.
5. Roberts HH. The therapeutic value of the spas and health resorts of America. Med Rec 1919;95:321.
6. Lowman CL. Technique of Underwater Gymnastics: A Study in Practical Application. Los Angeles: American Publications, 1937;4.
7. Conte RS. The History of the Greenbrier, America's Resort. Charlestown, WV: Pictorial Histories Publishing, 1989;121.
8. Cohen S. The Homestead and Warm Springs Valley, Virginia: A Pictorial Heritage. Charlestown, WV: Pictorial Histories Publishing, 1984;17.
9. Groedel FM. Memorial Meeting Bulletin. American College of Cardiology. October–November 1951.
10. Groedel FM. The Mineral Springs and Baths at Saratoga Springs. Saratoga, NY: Saratoga Springs Commission, 1932;2, 5.
11. McClellan WS. What is being done at New York state's great enterprise: Saratoga Springs. J Am Med Hydrology 1932;1:27.
12. Publications of Saratoga Spa, No. 1. Saratoga, NY: Saratoga Springs Authority, 1935.
13. The American Society of Medical Hydrology. Working Committee Minutes of Meeting Held at French Lick Springs Hotel. December 4, 1931. In the archives of The American Society of Medical Hydrology.
14. Coulter JS. Physical Therapy, Vol 7. The CLIO Medica Series of Primers on the History of Medicine. Chicago, 1932.
15. Wright R. Hydrotherapy in Psychiatric Hospitals. Boston: Tudor Press, 1940.
16. Martin LG. Under Water Physiotherapy and Pool Therapy. Presented with motion pictures before the 58th Annual Session of the Arkansas Medical Society at Hot Springs National Park, AR. May 2–4, 1933.
17. Smith EM. Hydrotherapy in Arthritis, Underwater Therapy Applied to Chronic Atrophic Arthritis. Presented before the 14th Annual Session of the American Congress of Physical Therapy, Kansas City, MO. September 11, 1935. Also presented at the Annual Meeting of the American Therapeutic Society, Atlantic City, NJ. June 4–5, 1937.
18. Fletcher GB. Underwater or Pool Treament of Certain Conditions of Muscles, Nerves and Joints. Read before the Tri-State Medical Society, Marshall, TX. November 9, 1939.
19. King N. Pool Therapy. Presented at the Garland County-Hot Springs Medical Society, Hot Springs, AR. January 12, 1932.
20. Wallace AW. The modern health resort, an appraisal of its possibilities. JAMA 1936;107:419.
21. Groedel FM. Physiologic effect of carbon-dioxide baths on the circulatory system. Arch Phys Ther X-ray Radium 1937;18:457.
22. McClellan WS. The Saratoga Spa, its place in the treatment of rheumatic disorders. Arch Phys Ther X-ray Radium 1937;18:468.
23. Behrend HJ. Modern hydrotherapy. Arch Phys Ther X-ray Radium 1937;18:146.
24. American health resorts [editorial]. Arch Phys Ther X-ray Radium 1937;18:509.
25. McClellan WS. A History of the American Spa. Mimeographed unpublished manuscript. 1959;11. Found at Hot Springs, AR, Library.
26. Fantus B. Our insufficiently appreciated American spas and health resorts. JAMA 1938;110:40.
27. McClellan WS. Unpublished program notes from 1938 Spa Inspection Tour of American Spas Committee.
28. McClellan WS. Report on spas and health resorts. Arch Phys Ther X-ray Radium 1937;20: 42, 52.

29. McClellan WS. Spas, American style. Med Econ 1939;(Oct):37.

30. Kovacs R. American spas. Med Rec 1941;153:254.

31. Sigerist HE. American spas in historical perspective. Bull Hist Med 1942;11:133.

32. McClellan WS. The utilization of health resorts for military reconstruction. JAMA 1943;123:564.

33. Sigerist HE. Towards a renaissance of the American spa. Ciba Found Symp 1946;8:333.

34. Cole A, Becker B. Introduction to aquatic rehabilitation. J Back Musculoskel Rehab 1994;4:7.

35. Henriksen JD. Spa cardiac rehabilitation. Med Hydrology Q 1969;1:1.

36. Burt B. Fodor's Health and Fitness Vacations. New York: Fodor's Travel Publications, 1989.

2

Biophysiologic Aspects of Hydrotherapy

Bruce E. Becker

It is not surprising that hydrotherapy, the therapeutic external use of water for medical purposes, was one of the earliest forms of rehabilitation. Water has always been ubiquitous, known to promote healing, and known to be useful to a broad range of medical ailments. As noted in Chapter 1, natural springs and water therapies became a central focus of many health-promoting establishments. Healers from all backgrounds have noted the effects of water on various medical problems. Through observation, centuries of trial and error, and scientific methodology, traditions of healing through aquatic treatments have evolved. Water has been found to exert a great many biological effects. Over recent decades, the therapeutic external application of water, usually through immersion of part or all of the body for the purpose of obtaining these biological effects came to be called *medical hydrology*.

Recent research into the rehabilitative aspects of aquatic therapies has been sparse. Were it not for two fortuitous aspects of aquatic immersion, very little current research would be available and the hapless practitioner would have to rely on the centuries of oral and written traditions for guidance, at the risk of being labeled an unscientific practitioner. The first fortunate stimulus for recent research was the recognition that aquatic immersion is an ideal method of studying cardiac, pulmonary, and renal responses to sudden changes in blood volume, an essential part of understanding how humans maintain normal function during physiologic change. The second circumstance was the recognition that aquatic immersion is an ideal environment to mimic weightlessness. As man prepared to enter the space environment, scientists needed to better understand the effects that space might have on the human organism. Critical basic science research was performed on essentially all biological systems under aquatic immersion, so that the necessary understanding of physiology could be gained in preparation for man's first true total escape from gravity. Thus, as we prepared to send man into space, the ultimate technologic environment, we found answers in what was our first environment: thermoneutral total body immersion. As a consequence of these two driving forces to understand human physiology, aquatic rehabilitation has a wealth of basic science research as a foundation, indeed a better and broader foundation than many other rehabilitative techniques.

Aquatic immersion has profound biological effects, extending across essentially all homeostatic systems. These effects are both immediate and delayed, and they allow water to be used with therapeutic efficacy for a great variety of rehabilitative problems. Aquatic therapies are beneficial in the management of patients with musculoskeletal problems, neurologic problems, cardiopulmonary pathology, and other conditions. In addition, the margin of therapeutic safety is wider than that of almost any other treatment milieu. Knowledge of these biological effects can aid the skilled rehabilitative clinician.

AQUATIC PHYSICS

Water is composed of oxygen and hydrogen. One atom of oxygen bonds with two atoms of hydrogen to form a molecule of water (H_2O) with a molecular weight of 18. The nearest approach of water molecules occurs in ice, in which state they are separated by 0.276 nm. The radius of the molecule is 0.138 nm. The molecules are bonded triangularly, with the hydrogen atoms separated by an arc of 104 degrees, 31 seconds, and separated from the oxygen atom by 0.0958 nm. This angle is greater than the expected 90 degrees because of the incomplete sharing of electrons between the oxygen and hydrogen atoms, creating a partially ionized state. The physical configuration of these bonded molecules creates an open electrical field, which creates affinity for many other chemical substances, hence water's tremendous solubility [1].

Matter commonly exists at normal Earth temperatures in three states: solid, liquid, and gas. A solid maintains a consistent shape and size, which typically does not change without significant force. In contrast, liquids readily alter shape but typically retain volume despite force. Gases are the least fixed, lacking a fixed shape and size. Both liquids and gases have the ability to flow, and because flow properties depend more on density than on any other factor, both are referred to as fluids. Although water is used in all its forms therapeutically, this chapter deals only with water in its liquid form.

Nearly all the biological effects of immersion are related to the fundamental principles of hydrodynamics. An understanding of these principles makes the medical application process more rational.

Static Properties of Water

Density and Specific Gravity

Density is defined as mass per unit volume, and is given the Greek letter ρ (rho) [2]. The relationship of ρ to mass and volume is characterized by the formula:

$$\rho = \frac{m}{V}$$

where m is the mass of a substance whose volume is V. Density is measured in the international system by kilograms per cubic meter and occasionally as grams per cubic centimeter. A density given in the latter format must be multiplied by 1,000 to equal the former. Density is a temperature-dependent variable, although this is much less so for solids and liquids than for gases. Water reaches its maximum density at 4°C. Water has the unusual property of becoming less dense below the freezing point; typically, as liquids freeze they become more dense. This property of water is important, because if water were typical, as it froze into ice, it would sink into the mass of still-liquid water, thus allowing lakes to freeze from the bottom, killing off most of the biomass within.

In addition to density, substances are defined by their specific gravity, the ratio of the density of that substance to the density of water. Water has a specific gravity equal to 1 at 4°C (because this number is a ratio, it has no units). Although the human body is mostly water, the body's density is slightly less than that of water and averages a specific gravity of 0.974, with males averaging higher density than females. Lean body mass, which includes bone, muscle, connective tissue, and organs, has a typical density near 1.1, whereas fat mass, which includes both essential body fat plus fat in excess of essential needs has a density of about 0.9 [3]. Highly fit and muscular males tend toward specific gravities greater than 1, whereas an unfit or obese male might be considerably less. Consequently, the human body displaces a volume of water weighing slightly more than the body, forcing the body upward by a force equal to the volume of the water displaced.

Hydrostatic Pressure

Pressure is defined as force per unit area, where the force, F, by convention is understood to act perpendicularly to the surface area, A. This relationship is expressed as:

$$P = \frac{F}{A}$$

The standard international unit of pressure is called a pascal, abbreviated Pa, after the French scientist Blaise Pascal, and is measured in newtons per square meter. Other common measurement units are dynes per square centimeter, kilograms per square meter, millimeters of mercury (mm Hg) per foot, and pounds per square inch (psi).

Fluids have been found experimentally to exert pressure in all directions, as swimmers and divers know. If a theoretic point is immersed in a vessel of water, the pressure exerted on that point is equal from all directions. If unequal pressure were being exerted, the point would move until the pressures on it were equalized.

Pressure in a liquid increases with depth and is directly related to the density of the fluid. If a theoretic point is immersed to a distance, h, below the surface, the force exerted on the point is due to the weight of the column of fluid above it. The formula F (force) = m (mass) × g (the acceleration of gravity) defines the force, and is equal to ρ (density) × A (area) × h (the height of the column of fluid). Thus, pressure is expressed as:

$$P = \frac{F}{A} = \frac{\rho A h g}{A}$$

By canceling out A, we find that

$$P = \rho g h$$

Therefore, pressure is directly proportional to both the liquid density and to the immersion depth when the fluid is incompressible, as water is at the depths used in therapeutic environments. Sometimes it is useful to know the pressure differential between two immersed points separated by a vertical distance, h. This pressure differential may be calculated by the adapted formula:

$$\Delta P = \rho g \Delta h$$

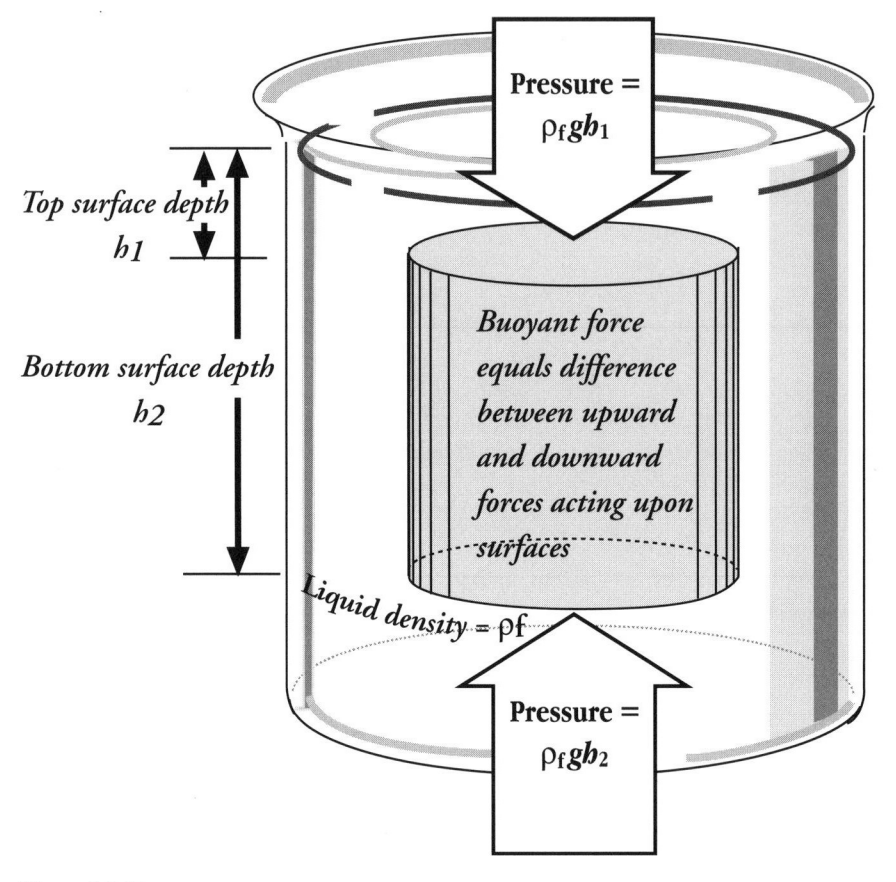

Top surface depth
$h1$

Bottom surface depth
$h2$

Pressure =
$\rho_f g h_1$

Buoyant force equals difference between upward and downward forces acting upon surfaces

Liquid density = ρ_f

Pressure =
$\rho_f g h_2$

Figure 2-1. Buoyancy.

where Δ is the change in pressure and depth. Because P responds not only to the fluid depth but also to any force exerted on its surface, the pressure of Earth's atmosphere is an important contributor to the total force from immersion. Water exerts a pressure of 22.4 mm Hg/ft of water depth, which translates to 1 mm Hg/1.36 cm (0.54 in.) of water depth. Thus a body immersed to a depth of 48 in. is subjected to a force equal to 88.9 mm Hg, which is slightly greater than diastolic blood pressure. This is the force that aids the resolution of edema in an injured body part.

Buoyancy

Immersed objects have less apparent weight than the same object on land because a force opposite to gravity is acting on the object. This force is called *buoyancy*, the upward force generated by the volume of water displaced. Buoyancy arises from the fact that pressure in a fluid increases with depth. A cylinder immersed vertically in water (Figure 2-1) has more force exerted on its bottom surface than on its top surface. A cylinder with height h has top and bottom surfaces with area A and is immersed in a liquid with density ρ_f. Because the pressure on the top of the cylinder is equal to $\rho_f g h_1$, where g is the force of gravity and h_1 is the top surface depth, the force developed is $F_1 = P_1 A$, which is equal to $\rho_f g h_1 A$ and is a downward force. A force pushing up on the bottom surface of the cylinder is calculated by similar means. This force equates to $F_2 = P_2 A = \rho_f g h_2 A$. The net force is called the *buoyant force* F_B, and it pushes up with the magnitude:

$$
\begin{aligned}
F_B &= F_2 - F_1 \\
&= \rho_f g A (h_2 - h_1) \\
&= \rho_f g A h \\
&= \rho_f g V
\end{aligned}
$$

where $V = Ah$ is the volume of the cylinder. Because ρ_f is the density of the liquid,

$$
\rho_f g V = m_f g
$$

defines the weight of fluid of comparable volume to the cylinder volume. Thus the buoyant force F_B is equal to the weight of the fluid displaced. This principle, discovered by Archimedes, explains why we float, why water can be used as a laboratory for weightlessness, and why water can be used to advantage in the management of medical problems requiring weight off-loading. The principle applies equally to floating objects. A human with specific gravity of 0.97 reaches floating equilibrium when 97% of his or her volume is submerged.

Center of Buoyancy vs. Center of Balance.   The product of a force and a distance over which the force acts is called a *moment*, and it may also be called *torque*. Although the terms are technically equivalent, *torque* is often used with reference to rotational motion. The fact that the force of buoyancy is an upward force leads to important consequences in the therapeutic aquatic environment. Center of gravity is a point at which all force moments (the magnitude of forces with their respective directions of action) are in equilibrium. For a human being standing in the anatomic position, the center of gravity is located slightly posterior to the midsagittal plane and at the level of the second sacral vertebra because the human body is not uniform with respect to density (e.g., the lungs are less dense than the lower limbs). The center of gravity is really the physical aggregate of the centers of gravity of all the body parts.

The center of buoyancy is defined as the center of all buoyancy force moments. Consequently, the human center of buoyancy is in the midchest (Figure 2-2). When both centers are aligned in a vertical plane, only vertical vector forces are apparent, which may produce a compressive or distractive force on the body. When these points are not aligned vertically, a rotational force results. This force is defined by the horizontal displacement of centers and the vector magnitude difference between the upward force on the center of buoyancy and the downward force on the center of gravity. This torque force may assist the floating human in maintaining an upright head-out posture, or, when buoyancy devices are used, may tend to float a person face down (supine). These same forces affect a limb and become a vector continuum as the limb moves through water.

Buoyancy and Joint Loading.   As the body is gradually immersed, water is displaced, creating the force of buoyancy. This takes the weight off the immersed joints progressively, and with neck immersion, only about 15 lbs of compressive

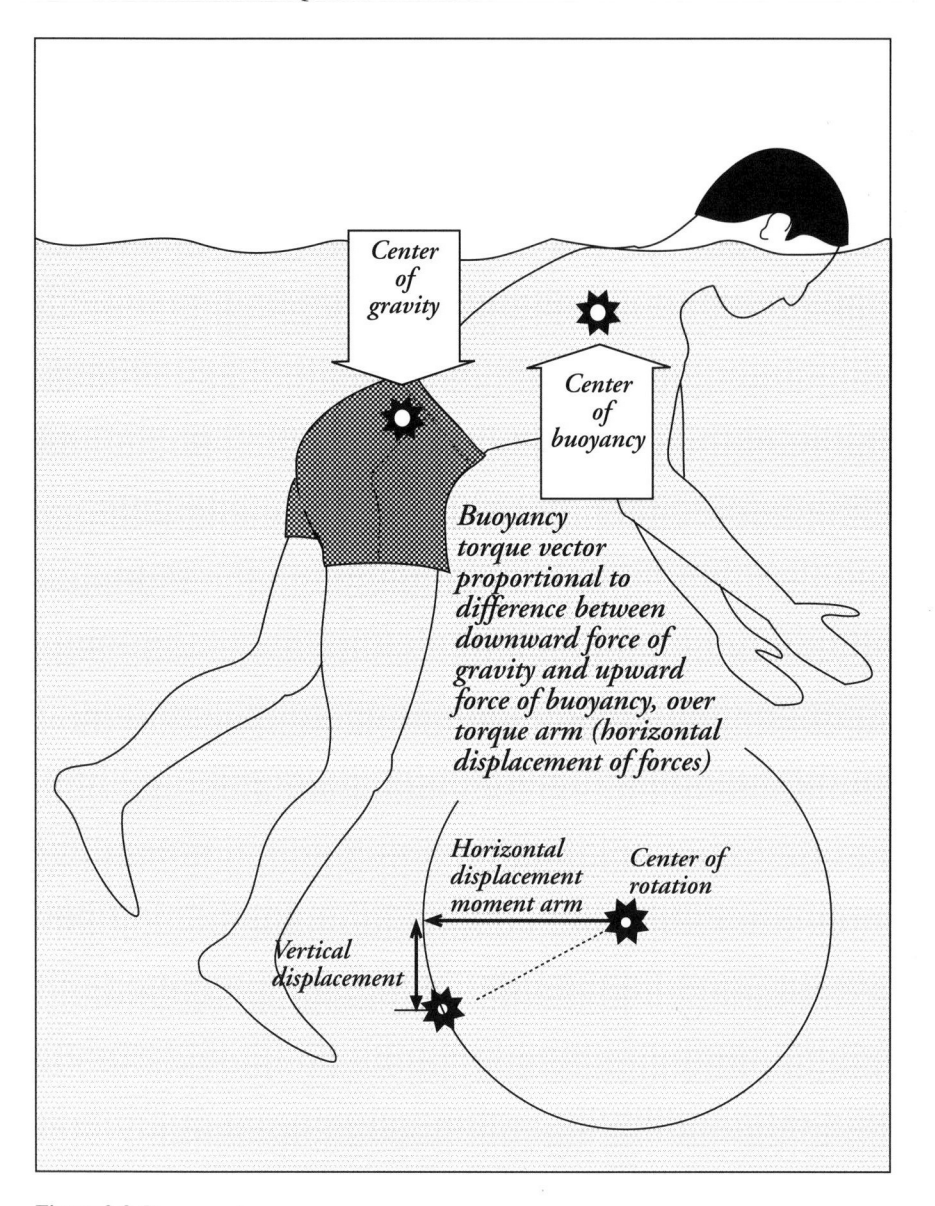

Figure 2-2. Buoyancy torque.

force (the approximate weight of the head) is exerted on the spine, hips, and knees. A person immersed to the symphysis pubis has effectively off-loaded 40% of his or her body weight, and when further immersed to the umbilicus, approximately 50%. Xiphoid immersion off-loads body weight by 60% or more, depending on whether the arms are overhead or beside the trunk. A body suspended or floating in water essentially counterbalances the downward effects of gravity with the upward force of buoyancy. This effect may be of great therapeutic utility. For example, a fractured pelvis may not become mechanically stable under full body loading for a period of many weeks, but with water immersion, gravitational forces may be partially or completely offset so that only muscle torque forces act on the fracture site, allowing active assisted range-of-motion activities, gentle strength building, and even gait training.

Refraction

When light passes from one medium to another, it encounters a boundary layer and generally undergoes a change at this interface. Part of the incident light is reflected at the boundary, and the portion passing into the new medium may change direction. This bending is referred to as *refraction* and is governed by specific properties of the material, particularly the speed of light in the material, and the angle of incidence of the light beam. This phenomenon was studied in the early 1600s by Willebrord Snell, who discovered a consistent relationship between θ (theta), the angle of incidence, and n, the index of refraction. This relationship, called *Snell's law*, is expressed as follows:

$$n_1 \sin\theta_1 = n_2 \sin\theta_2$$

where θ_1 is the angle of incidence, θ_2 is the angle of refraction, and n_1 and n_2 are the respective indices of refraction in air and water, respectively. Thus, if light enters a medium in which n is greater (and speed is less), the beam of light is bent toward the normal (perpendicular to the interface). Conversely, when light exiting a medium of high n enters a medium of low n, such as air, it deviates from the normal.

Consequently, from the pool edge, a person standing in waist-deep water appears to have foreshortened trunk and legs, and this foreshortening increases with the distance from the observer to the immersed person, given that both are on the same plane, as the angle of the incident light θ increases. In a therapeutic environment, it requires experience and careful attention to recognize the difference between the appearance of a body part location and its true position.

Surface Tension

The surface of a liquid acts like a membrane under tension. Thus, a drop of water may hang on the end of a straw, and a needle heavier than water may float on the surface of a glass of water, suspended from this membrane-like barrier. This is because the attraction between adjacent molecules of water is circumferential everywhere except at the surface, where the attraction bonding is parallel to the surface. Surface tension is defined as the force F per unit length L that acts across any line in a surface and tends to pull the surface open [2]. Surface tension is denoted by the Greek letter γ (gamma), and the force equation is

$$\gamma = \frac{F}{L}$$

Work must be done to increase the surface area of the fluid. Consequently, in absence of a force input, fluids tend to be shaped in ways that minimize the surface area. A raindrop assumes a shape that offers the minimum surface area consistent with the drop's volume, speed, and temperature.

Time-Dependent Properties of Water

Water in Motion

Water in motion is a complex physical substance. In fact, despite centuries of study, many aspects of fluid motion are still incompletely understood. The major principles of flow are known and can be applied to general activities.

Flow Motion

Water in motion has several characteristics. When water moves smoothly, with all layers moving at the same speed, the water is said to be in *laminar* or *streamline flow*. In this type of movement, all molecules are moving parallel to each other and their paths do not cross. Typically, laminar flow rates are slow because when water moves rapidly even minor oscillations create uneven flow and parallel paths are knocked out of alignment. When this latter condition occurs another type of pattern develops, called *turbulent flow*. In turbulent flow, flow patterns arise that run dramatically out of parallel and may even set up paths running in opposite directions. These paths, called *eddy currents*, look like whirlpools in response to obstacles in the flow path or to irregularities in the surface of flow-directing vessels. Examples of irregularities are the eddy holes that appear behind boulders in fast-moving streams and eddy currents that form in the bloodstream inside arteries encrusted with cholesterol plaque. Turbulent flow absorbs energy at a much greater rate than streamline flow, and the rate of energy absorption is determined by the internal friction in the fluid. This internal friction is called viscosity. The major determinants of water motion are viscosity, turbulence, and speed.

Viscosity.   Water at room temperature and through most of the range of its commonest therapeutic uses is a liquid. Liquids share a property called *viscosity*, which refers to the magnitude of internal friction specific to the fluid. Different fluids possess varying amounts of molecular attraction within the fluid, and as layers of fluid are set into motion, this attraction creates resistance to movement and is detected as friction. Energy must be exerted to create movement, and, as in the first law of thermodynamics, energy is never lost but rather transformed and stored as potential or kinetic energy. Some energy is transformed into heat, some into kinetic energy, and some may be stored as energy by increasing surface tension. Fluids are in part defined by individual viscosity, expressed quantitatively as the coefficient of viscosity, which is designated by the Greek letter η (eta). The greater the coefficient, the more viscous the fluid and the more force is required to create movement within the fluid. This force is proportionate to the number of molecules of fluid set in motion and the velocity of their movement. Because velocity is described as distance over time, viscosity is the first time-dependent property of water. Thus, the equation that expresses this relationship must define the volume of the fluid in motion (F), where A is the area, l is depth, and v is the velocity of the motion:

$$F = \eta \, A \frac{v}{l}$$

Table 2-1. Coefficients of Viscosities for a Variety of Fluids

Fluid	Temperature (°C)	Coefficient of Viscosity η (Pa·s)
Water	0	1.8×10^{-3}
Whole blood	37	4×10^{-3}
Blood plasma	37	1.5×10^{-3}
Engine oil (SAE 10)	30	200×10^{-3}
Glycerin	20	$1,500 \times 10^{-3}$
Water vapor	100	0.013×10^{-3}

Pa·s = Pascal seconds.

Solving this equation for η finds that $\eta = Fl/vA$. The standard international unit of measurement of viscosity is measured in newton seconds/m^2 (this is equivalent to a pascal-second (Pa·s). In the centimeters/gram/second (cgs) system, the measurement is dyne-seconds/cm^2. One unit is called a *poise*, after the French scientist J.L. Poiselle (1799–1869), who studied the physics of blood circulation. Often, coefficients are stated in centipoise (one-hundredth of a poise) (Table 2-1).

Laminar Flow.   As water moves smoothly within a vessel, the speed of movement changes with the size of the vessel. The flow rate is defined as the mass of water (m) moving past an imaginary point per a unit of time t: m/t.

$$\frac{\Delta m}{\Delta t} = \frac{\rho_1 \Delta V_1}{\Delta t} = \frac{\rho_1 A_1 l_1}{\Delta t} = \rho_1 A_1 v_1$$

where ρ_1 represents fluid density at a point in space 1, V_1 represents the volume of water, v_1 the velocity of flow, and l_1 the length of water column of area A_1. As water moves past a subsequent point 2, the same volume of water with area A_2 and length l_2 may need to increase or decrease velocity to adapt to vessel area changes because water is essentially incompressible.

Poiselle developed an equation that describes the laminar flow of an incompressible fluid through a tube of fixed internal radius and length.

$$Q = \frac{\pi R^4 (P_1 - P_2)}{8 \eta L}$$

Q (the volume rate of flow) is directly proportional to the pressure gradient and inversely proportional to the viscosity and is also proportional to the fourth power of the tube radius. Therefore, if the tube doubles in radius, flow volume increases by a factor of 16. This equation only holds true for laminar flow, however, and only provides an approximation of turbulent flow volumes.

Turbulent Flow.   Flow volumes lessen when turbulence occurs, largely due to the significant rise in internal friction in the fluid. The onset of turbulent flow is a function of fluid velocity, but it is also related to fluid density, viscosity, and enclosure radius. Laminar flow is compared with turbulent flow in Figure 2-3. The transition

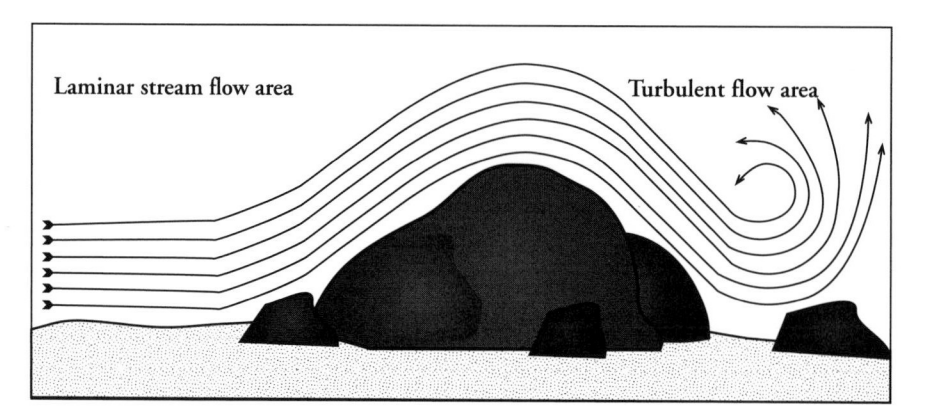

Figure 2-3. Laminar and turbulent flow.

from laminar to turbulent flow often occurs abruptly. This transition point is characterized by a formula incorporating these factors and is called the *Reynolds number* (Re), after the English physicist Sir Joshua Reynolds. This number is calculated by the formula:

$$Re = \frac{2\tilde{v}r\rho}{\eta}$$

where $\tilde{v}$ is the average fluid velocity, ρ is fluid density, and r the radius of the tube in which the fluid is flowing. Typically, Reynolds numbers greater than 2,000 produce turbulent flow.

Drag Contribution

When an object moves relative to a fluid, it is subjected to the resistive effects of the fluid. This force is called *drag force* and is due to fluid viscosity and turbulence when present. This force is defined by a second Reynolds number:

$$Re' = \frac{vL\rho}{\eta}$$

where v equals the velocity of the object relative to the fluid. Although the Reynolds formulas are similar, the results are different. A 1-mm object moving through water at 1 mm per second has a Reynolds number of 1. When this formula produces a Reynolds number equal to or less than 1, the flow is usually laminar, and the force needed to move through the fluid is directly proportional to the speed of the object. The viscous force F_v is directly proportional to the object speed:

$$F_v = kv$$

where k is the second Reynolds number. The magnitude of k depends on the size and shape of the object and on the fluid viscosity. If the object is a sphere, this k is equal to

$$k = 6\pi r\eta$$

With faster movement, higher Reynolds numbers are produced, and the drag force begins to increase as the square of the velocity. The force required to move through water thus becomes

$$F_d = kv^2$$

where F_d is drag force and k is the Reynolds number. Streamlining reduces the resultant Reynolds number. The speed needed to produce Reynolds numbers between 1 and 10 produces turbulence behind the object, known as a *wake*. At these speeds, the force increases with the square of the velocity, $F_v \propto v^2$. As the speed increases yet further, with Reynolds numbers around 106, there is an abrupt increase in drag force. This force is due to turbulence produced not only behind the moving object but also in the layer of fluid passing over the object, known as the *boundary layer*.

Resistance Effects

Water is intermediate in viscosity as liquids go, but it still presents much resistance to movement. Under turbulent flow conditions, this resistance increases as a log function of velocity and depends on the shape and size of the object. The greatest surface area drag in a swimming person is the head, although the negative pressure following the swimmer causes the greatest force resisting forward movement. There is turbulence produced by the moving body surface areas, and a drag force produced by the turbulence behind. Viscosity, with all its attendant physical properties, is a quality that makes water a useful strengthening medium. Viscous resistance increases as more force is exerted against it, but that resistance drops to zero almost immediately on cessation of force because there is only a small amount of inertial moment. (Viscosity effectively counteracts inertial momentum.) Thus, when a rehabilitating person feels pain and stops movement, the force drops precipitously and water viscosity damps movement almost instantaneously. This allows great control of strengthening activities within the envelope of patient comfort.

Because much aquatic rehabilitation usefulness comes from the movement of a person through water, it is worth understanding the variables involved in propulsion. The work involved in overcoming drag force equals the product of the magnitude of the drag force times the displacement. Because drag depends on the square of the velocity, w_d, the work done in joules equals

$$w_d = F_d d = kv^2 d$$

where d equals the displacement, k the Reynolds number, and v the velocity. Power refers to work done per unit time. In this instance, the power to overcome drag, P_d, equals the drag force times the velocity, and thus,

$$P_d = F_d v = kv^3$$

so that the power to overcome drag at a given speed depends on the Reynolds factor and the cube of the velocity. In water walking, a person can use ground reaction forces to move forward, and thus inertia and viscous resistance are the essential factors. In swimming, propulsion depends on thrust, which is achieved through attempting to propel water backward, thus gaining forward movement according to Newton's third law of motion: To every action there is an equal and opposite reaction. The mass of water propelled backward (m_1) is given a velocity change (Δv_i)

and thus an impulse equal to $m_1\Delta v_i$. Because this happens in stroke-by-stroke and kick-by-kick increments, the mean propulsive force equals:

$$F_p = \int_0^T F_p\, dt = \frac{1}{T}\Sigma m_i \cdot v_i$$

where F_p equals the force of propulsion, d equals displacement, and T equals time. The swimmer must not only transfer kinetic energy to the water through this change in velocity of the water but must also exert energy to overcome drag. Of course, the energy translated to the water being accelerated is lost to propulsion of the swimmer. Because water is viscous and resists with the log of velocity, with increasing swim effort, less energy may be wasted on water acceleration and more used on swimmer propulsion. Alas, with increasing swim speed, turbulent drag increases. The net effect is that stroke efficiency may increase at rapid speeds, but this efficiency is expended in overcoming drag.

THERMODYNAMICS OF WATER

Specific Heat

Water is used therapeutically in all its thermal forms: solid, liquid, and gas. A major reason for its usefulness lies in the physics of aquatic thermodynamics. All substances on earth possess energy stored as heat. This energy is measured in a quantity called a *calorie*, abbreviated *cal*. A calorie is defined as the heat required to raise the temperature of 1 g water by 1°C, for example, from 14.5°C to 15.5°C. The energy required to raise the temperature of water varies slightly, even though this difference is less than 1% in the range of 0–100°C. Sometimes the energy required to raise temperature is defined in kilocalories, the amount required to raise 1 kilogram of water by 1°C. This unit by convention is termed a *Calorie* (with a capital C), abbreviated *Cal*. This is the unit in which food energy content is measured. The British system measures heat energy in British thermal units (BTU), the amount of energy required to raise 1 lb of water by 1°F. A mass of water possesses a definable, measurable amount of stored energy in the form of heat.

The amount of energy stored may be released in change to a lower temperature, or additional energy may be required to raise temperature. The formula defining the quantity of energy required or released is

$$Q = mc\Delta T$$

where m equals the mass of water, c equals the specific heat capacity of the fluid, and ΔT equals the change in temperature. The work required to produce this energy is called the *mechanical equivalent of heat*, and is measured in joules (J). One calorie is equivalent to 4.18 J. A body immersed in a mass of water becomes a dynamic system. If the temperature of the water exceeds the temperature of the submerged body, the system equilibrates to a different level, with the submerged body warming through transference of heat energy from the water, and the water cooling through loss of heat energy to the body. By the first law of thermodynamics, the total heat (and thus energy) content of the system remains the same. Energy applied to this system raises the kinetic energy of some of the molecules, and when high–kinetic-energy molecules collide with lower–kinetic-energy molecules, they transfer some of their energy, raising and equilibrating the total energy of the system.

Table 2-2. Various Heat Capacities

Substance	Specific Heat c_p
Water (15°C)	1.00
Ice (−5°C)	0.50
Steam (110°C)	0.48
Ethyl alcohol	0.58
Protein	0.40
Human body (avg.)	0.83
Mercury	0.033
Air	0.001

Again, by cgs system definition, water is defined as having a specific heat capacity equal to 1. In contrast, air has a significantly lower specific heat capacity (0.001). Thus, water retains heat 1,000 times more than an equivalent volume of air does (Table 2-2).

Thermal Energy Transfer

The therapeutic utility of water depends greatly on both its ability to retain heat and its ability to transfer heat energy. Exchange of energy in the form of heat occurs in three ways: (1) conduction, (2) convection, and (3) radiation. Conduction may be thought of as occurring through molecular collisions over a small distance. Convection requires the mass movement of large numbers of molecules over a large distance. Liquids and gases are generally poor conductors but good convectors. Radiation transfers heat through the transmission of electromagnetic waves. Conduction and convection require contact between the exchanging energy sources. Radiation does not. Conduction occurs in the absence of movement, but convection requires that energy transfer occurs through movement of one source across the other. The rate of radiant energy transfer from a body is proportional to the fourth power of its temperature in degrees Kelvin. It is also proportional to surface area, to the emissivity of the material, and to the distance between the energy-radiating and energy-absorbing bodies.

Heat transfer across a gradient is measured by the amount of heat in calories transferred per second across an imaginary membrane. Substances vary widely in their ability to conduct heat. Water is an efficient conductor, transferring heat 25 times faster than air.

Metals and water tend to conduct heat well, and gas or gas-containing materials (e.g., cork, glass, wool, and down) conduct heat poorly (Table 2-3). The latter are thus good insulators, whereas the former are good conductors. Human tissue without blood is a rather good insulator.

The human body produces considerable heat through the conversion of food calories into other energy forms. Only about 20% of this converted energy is used to do work, and the rest is converted into thermal energy. Core temperature would rise about 3°C per hour during light activity if not for the body's ability to dissipate heat. This dissipation process occurs through all heat transfer mechanisms, but by far the most important is convection, occurring through the flow of warm blood from the core to the skin and lungs, where contact with the cooler air occurs. Blood becomes

Table 2-3. Thermal Conductivity

Substance	Thermal Conductivity (k) (kcal/sec/m/°C)
Water (15°C)	1.4×10^{-4}
Air	0.055×10^{-4}
Human tissue (bloodless)	0.5×10^{-4}
Glass	2.0×10^{-4}
Silver	10×10^{-2}
Copper	9.2×10^{-2}
Down	0.06×10^{-4}
Cork and glass wool	0.1×10^{-4}

a convective fluid that transfers heat to the surface. Because energy must be further dissipated, the body uses another mechanism, which allows energy loss through the latent heat of evaporation of sweat and respiratory loss, further cooling the skin. This mechanism is remarkably efficient because the evaporative loss of 2.5 ml of water cools the body 0.94°C (2°F). This fact is of considerable importance in scuba diving, where the humidity of inspired air approaches 0% humidity, and the temperature of surrounding water is always lower than that of the diver's body [4]. Consequently, even in warm ocean waters, the diver sustains significant heat loss through respiratory evaporative water loss, dropping core temperature in a short period of time. Typically, the compensatory mechanism used is the wet suit, to insulate against heat loss through the skin, even though the respiratory loss cannot be prevented.

Heat transfer increases as a function of velocity. Thus, a swimmer loses more heat when swimming rapidly through cold water than does a person standing still in the same water. Fortunately for the swimmer, heat is produced through exercise. Heat transfer is achieved through all three mechanisms: conduction, convection, and radiation with transfer to an immersed human body mostly occurring through conduction and convection, though heat loss from the body to the surrounding water occurs mostly through radiation and convection. This thermal conductive property, in combination with the high specific heat of water, makes the use of water in rehabilitation very versatile because water retains heat or cold while delivering it easily to the immersed body part.

These physiologic effects start immediately on immersion. Heat transfer begins, and as the specific heat of the human body is less than that of water, the body equilibrates faster than water does. Hydrostatic pressure effects begin immediately, although most of these effects are to cause plastic deformation of the body through time (for example, blood displaces cephalad, right atrial pressure begins to rise, pleural surface pressure rises, the chest wall compresses, and the diaphragm is displaced cephalad).

FUNDAMENTAL BIOLOGICAL ASPECTS OF AQUATIC THERAPY

Circulatory System

Water exerts pressure on the immersed body. The column of blood contained in the arterial system is under pressure generated by the left ventricle during systolic contraction, and normal blood pressure at rest is less than 130 mm Hg. Blood remains under pressure during diastole, the period of ventricular relaxation, because of the closure of the mitral valve, and the elastic properties of the arterial system sustain the pressure at 60–70 mm Hg on average in the normotensive adult. The diastolic pressure is largely determined by the autonomic nervous system–controlled peripheral vascular tree through smooth muscle within the vessel walls, creating peripheral resistance.

Pressure in the venous side of the circulation is much lower than pressure on the arterial side of the system. Venous pressures vary depending on the part of the body and its vertical relationship to the heart. Venous pressures are in part controlled by the system of valves, which prevent backflow. These one-way valves act to divide the large vertical column of venous blood into many short columns with little vertical height. These valves create much lower hydrostatic pressure gradients inside the vein and shorten the effective fluid column so that the maximum venous pressure is 30 mm Hg peripherally, decreasing steadily so that blood reaching the right atrium has a negative pressure (–2 to –4 mm Hg). The role of these valves in maintaining a low-pressure system is critical, as can be observed when they fail, creating venous varicosities due to the lack of sufficient vessel wall strength to support the increased fluid column. This low-pressure gradient system that exists within the venous system is the driving force returning blood to the heart. Consequently, venous return is very sensitive to external pressure changes, including compression from surrounding muscles, and certainly from external water pressure. Because an individual immersed in water is subjected to external water pressure in a gradient, which within a relatively small depth exceeds venous pressure, blood is displaced upward through this one-way system, first into the thighs, then into the abdominal cavity vessels, and finally into the great vessels of the chest cavity and into the heart. Venous return is enhanced by the shift of blood from the periphery to trunk vessels to thorax to heart. Central venous pressure begins to rise with immersion to the xiphoid and increases until the body is completely immersed. Right atrial pressure increases by 14–18 mm Hg with immersion to the neck, going from about –2 to –4 mm Hg to 14–17 mm Hg [5,6]. When the whole body is immersed to the neck, the transmural pressure gradient of the right atrium increases significantly, measured by Arborelius et al. at 13 mm Hg, going from 2 to 15 mm Hg. Extra systoles may result, especially early in immersion [5].

Pulmonary blood flow increases with increased central blood volume and pressure. Mean pulmonary artery wedge pressure increases from 5 mm Hg on land to 22 mm Hg during immersion to the neck [5]. Most of the increased pulmonary blood volume is distributed in the larger vessels of the pulmonary vascular bed, and only a small percentage (≤5%), is at the capillary level. This is validated by the fact that the diffusion capacity of the lungs changes very little.

Central blood volume increased by 0.7 liter during immersion to the neck when studied by the Arborelius group [5]. This represents a 60% increase in central volume, with one-third of this volume taken up by the heart and the remainder by the great vessels of the lungs. Cardiac volume increases 27–30% with immersion to the neck [6]. But the heart is not a static receptacle. The healthy cardiac response to increased volume (stretch) is to increase force of contraction. As the myocardium stretches, an improved actin-myosin filament relationship is produced, enhancing the myocardial efficiency [7]. This increase in myocardial efficiency has been researched for nearly 70 years and is commonly referred to as *Starling's law*. Stroke volume increases as a result of this increased stretch. Although normal resting stroke

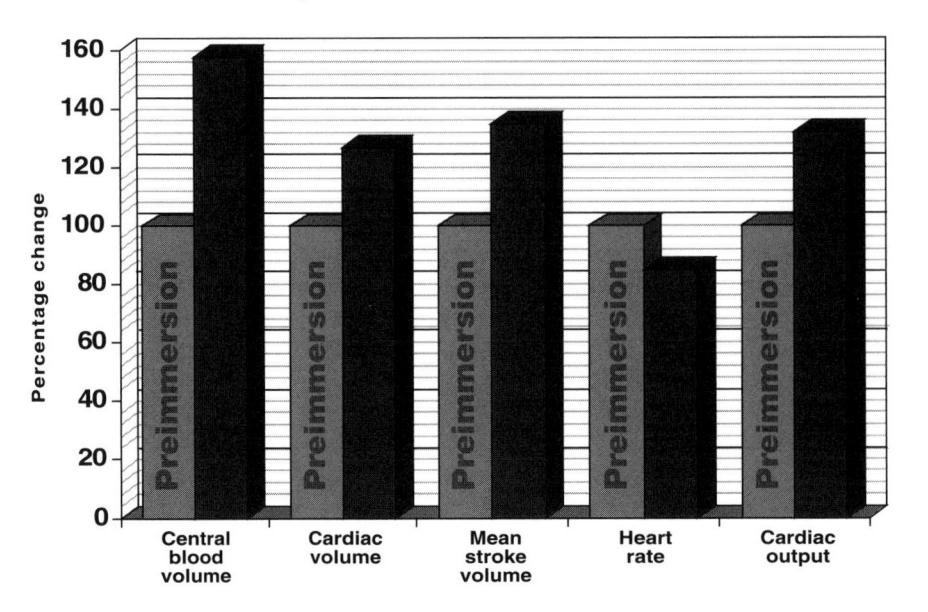

Figure 2-4. Cardiovascular changes following immersion.

volume is about 71 ml/beat, the additional 25 ml resulting from immersion equals about 100 ml, which is close to the exercise maximum for a sedentary deconditioned individual on land [8]. Mean stroke volume thus increases 35% on average with immersion to the neck [5]. There is both an increase in end-diastolic volume and a decrease in end-systolic volume [5]. These changes are compared to preimmersion status in Figure 2-4.

Most of the changes are temperature dependent, with cardiac output rising progressively with increasing water temperatures. Weston et al. found cardiac output to increase by 30% at 33°C and up to 121% at 39°C [7]. There is considerable individual variance in the many studies assessing this phenomenon.

Stroke volume is one of the major determinants of the rise in cardiac output seen with training; heart rate response ranges remain relatively fixed [8]. In an untrained individual, maximum heart rate is commonly approximated by subtracting the individual's age from a pulse rate of 200 beats per minute (bpm). The upper limit in an untrained individual is only 10–15% less than that in a trained one. As heart rate increases beyond an optimal point, cardiac output begins to decrease due to shortening of the diastole, which reduces time for ventricular filling as well as reducing time for coronary blood flow in the left ventricle circulatory tree [8]. Maximum stroke volume is reached at 40–50% of maximum oxygen consumption, which equals a heart rate of 110–120 bpm on land. This is generally accepted as the rate at which aerobic training begins [9].

As cardiac filling and stroke volume increase with progress in immersion depth from symphysis to xiphoid, the heart rate typically drops [10]. This drop is variable, with the amount of decrease dependent on water temperature. Typically, at average pool temperatures the rate lowers by 12–15% [6]. There is a significant relationship between water temperature and heart rate. At 25°C, heart rate drops approximately 12–15 bpm [11], whereas at thermoneutral temperatures, the rate drop is less than 15%, and in warm water, rate generally rises significantly, contributing to the major rise in cardiac output at high temperatures [7,12]. The reduction variability is related to decreased peripheral resistance at higher temperatures and increased vagal effects. A proposed diving response may be involved as well in colder temperatures.

Water-based exercise has often been said to be less effective than land-based exercise for improving cardiovascular fitness. Yet during exercise, maximal myocardial oxygen consumption efficiency (peak heart muscle efficiency) occurs with stroke volume increase because heart rate rise is a less efficient means of increasing output [7,8]. Stated another way, the most efficient way for the heart to deliver more blood is to increase stroke volume, as heart rate increase places greater demands on myocardium. Energy is wasted at the onset of myocardial contraction, when the heart is contracting but moving no volume, and at the endpoint of contraction, when the heart is moving little volume and the myocardium is maximally contracted. The optimal length-tension relationship develops with increased stroke volume. Thus, as cardiovascular conditioning occurs, cardiac output increases are achieved with smaller increases in heart rate but greater stroke volumes. This is the reason that conditioned athletes are able to maintain lower resting pulses while maintaining similar cardiac outputs compared to matched deconditioned individuals.

Two studies have validated the use of aquatic environments in cardiovascular rehabilitation following infarct and ischemic cardiomyopathy [13,14]. Both investigators took the bold step of actively rehabilitating patients with cardiac disease in an aquatic environment. Tanaka and Tei found that a single immersion in a very hot water (41°C) bath dropped both pulmonary wedge pressure and right atrial pressure by nearly 30%, and, over a period of 1 month of therapy, patients showed nearly a 30% rise in ejection fraction, significantly improving by one and sometimes two New York Heart Association classifications [14].

Cardiac output is the product of stroke volume times pulse rate per unit time. Because the ultimate purpose of the heart as an organ is to pump blood, its ultimate measure of performance is the amount of blood pumped per unit time. Immersion to the neck increases cardiac output by more than 30% [5]. Output increases by about 1,500 ml per minute, of which 50% is directed to increased muscle blood flow [6]. Normal cardiac output averages approximately 5 liters per minute in a resting individual. In a conditioned athlete, maximum output during very strenuous exercise is about 40 liters per minute, which is equivalent to 205 ml/beat times 195 bpm. Maximum output at exercise for a sedentary individual on land is approximately 20 liters per minute, which is equivalent to 105 ml/beat times 195 bpm [8]. Because immersion to the neck produces a cardiac stroke volume of about 100 ml/beat, a resting pulse of 86 bpm produces a cardiac output of 8.6 liters per minute and is already producing cardiac exercise. The increase in cardiac output appears to be somewhat age dependent, with younger subjects demonstrating greater increases (up 59%) than older subjects (up only 22%) [15]. The increase is also highly temperature dependent, varying directly with temperature increase, from 30% at 33°C to 121% at 39°C [16]. Research has shown that conditioned athletes demonstrate an even greater increase in cardiac output than untrained control subjects during immersed exercise and that this increase is sustained for longer periods than in the untrained control group [17]. Therefore, the myth that water exercise is not aerobically efficient is faulty: In fact, it may be an ideal cardiovascular conditioning medium. There is an emerging body of direct research data on water exercise–produced cardiac output but significant work needs to be done to delineate the effects of age, gender, temperature, and conditioning and to explain the significant individual response variations. The total cascade of cardiovascular responses is summarized in Figure 2-5.

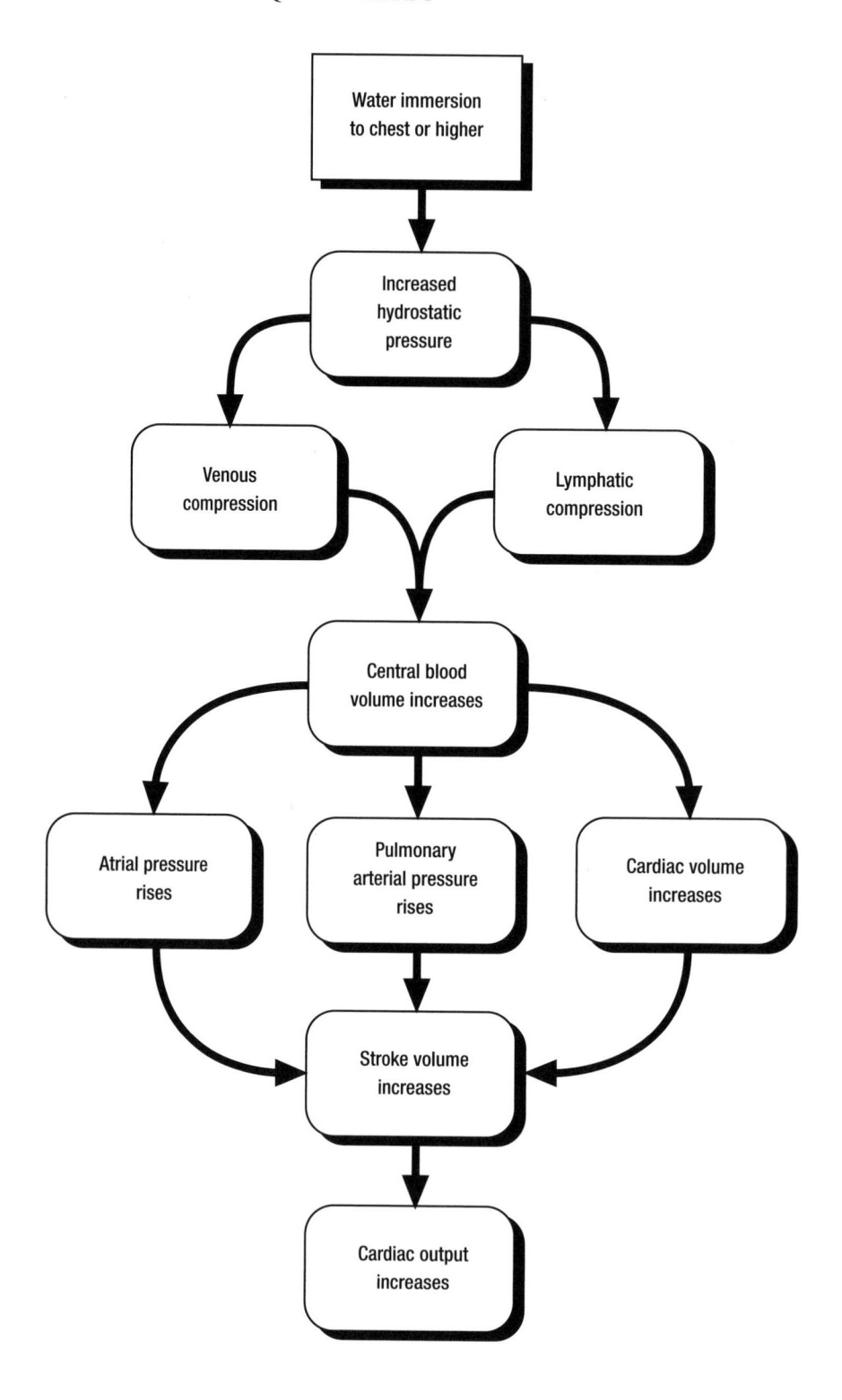

Figure 2-5. Schematic of cardiovascular changes following immersion.

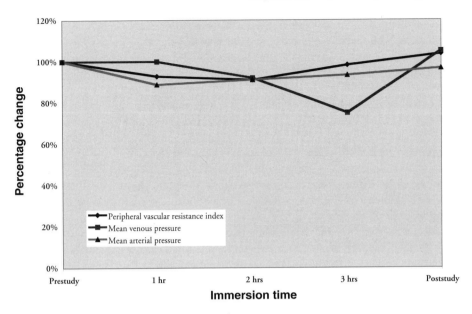

Figure 2-6. Vascular pressures during immersion.

It is possible to measure the actual resistance seen by the left ventricle. This resistance derives from the formula $P_{sa} - P_{ra}/Q$, where P_{sa} is the mean arterial pressure, P_{ra} is the mean right atrial pressure, and Q is cardiac output. During immersion to the neck, systemic vascular resistance decreases by 30% [5]. Decreased sympathetic vasoconstriction produces this decrease, with peripheral venous tone diminishing by 30%, from 17 to 12 mm Hg at thermoneutral temperatures [18]. Total peripheral resistance lowers during the first hour of immersion and persists for a period of hours thereafter. This drop is related to temperature, with higher temperatures producing greater drops. This decreases end-diastolic pressures. Systolic pressures increase with increasing workload but appear to be approximately 20% less in water than on land [7]. Venous pressures also drop during immersion because less vascular tone is required to support the system. These vascular pressure responses to immersion are demonstrated in Figure 2-6. Much study has been done on the effect of immersion on blood pressure. Very short–term immersion (10 minutes) in thermoneutral temperatures has been found to very slightly increase both systolic and diastolic pressures, perhaps as part of the cool water accommodation process [5]. Other studies done in carefully controlled environments have found no effects or actual drops in pressures. In an important study for aquatic rehabilitation, Coruzzi et al. found that longer immersion produced significant decreases in mean arterial pressure, with group I (sodium-sensitive) hypertensive patients showing even greater drops (–18 to –20 mm Hg) than normotensive patients, and group II (sodium-insensitive) patients smaller drops (–5 to –14 mm Hg) [19]. No studies have demonstrated consistent sustained increases in systolic pressure with prolonged immersion, although several have found no significant decreases. Based on a substantial body of research, the therapeutic pool appears to be a safe and potentially therapeutic environment for both normotensive and hypertensive patients, in contrast to widespread belief.

In 1989, Gleim and Nicholas found that oxygen consumption ($\dot{V}O_2$) was three times greater at a given speed of running (53 m/min) in water than on land [20].

Thus, looking at the reverse effect, during water walking and running, only one-half to one-third the speed was required to achieve the same metabolic intensity as on land [9]. It is important to note that the relationship of heart rate to $\dot{V}O_2$ during water exercise parallels that of land-based exercise, though water heart rate averages 10 bpm less, for reasons discussed earlier [5]. Consequently, metabolic intensity in water, as on land, may be predicted from monitoring heart rate.

Relative Perceived Exertion Scales

For more than 30 years it has been recognized that the subjective experience of effort is closely related to measurable parameters of workload. Through these years, beginning with the groundbreaking work of Gunnar Borg [21] and later confirmed by many other researchers, this relationship has been carefully studied. It is now known that the inner perception of effort closely correlates with $\dot{V}O_2$, blood and muscle lactate, heart rate, and other objective measurements. Coefficients of correlation with heart rates have ranged from 0.8 to 0.9, and high levels have also been shown with all other measures of exertion. It is significant that relative perceived exertion (RPE) scores correlate closely with blood lactate [22].

RPE scoring originated with Borg, who designed a rating scale to allow an individual to relate his or her effort level to a specific scale point, facilitating training consistency and measurement [21]. This scale used values ranging from 6 to 20 and was intended to represent pulse rate increase, with average resting pulse rate at 60 bpm, increasing to 200 bpm at maximum effort. Thus, a scale measurement was approximately equal to the heart rate divided by 10, although this numeric relationship should not be taken as sacred because many other variables affect heart rate on an individual basis. Borg cautioned against the use of RPE scales in cardiac rehabilitation settings because they had not been developed in the setting of known cardiac pathology. This scale has been modified in a number of ways by many, including Borg himself, who subsequently changed to a 10-point scale [23]. This 10-point scale has been successfully used in the aquatic environment by many practitioners. It has been found that the metabolic costs of aqua running are slightly less than treadmill running for equal RPE scores [24]. Wilder and Brennan developed a variant of the Borg scale for water-running exercise programs [25]: Their scale goes from 1 (light work) to 5 (extremely hard work).

Pulmonary System

The pulmonary system is profoundly affected by immersion of the body to the level of the thorax. Part of the effect is due to shifting of blood into the chest cavity, and part is due to compression of the chest wall itself by water. The combined effect is to alter pulmonary function, increase the work of breathing, and change respiratory dynamics.

A brief overview of pulmonary physiology aids understanding of the changes involved. When an individual is at rest, breathing comfortably, the normal excursion of air during inspiration and expiration is called *tidal volume*. At the endpoint of nonforced expiration, a volume of air remains in the lungs that can be expelled with increased effort. This volume is called *expiratory reserve volume* (ERV). ERV can be experienced by simply exhaling normally and then exhaling forcibly to the

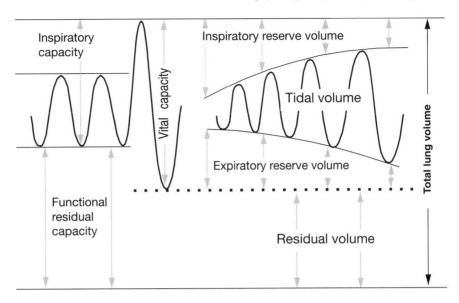

Figure 2-7. Pulmonary function divisions.

maximum amount. Even when this last volume has been expelled, air remains in the lungs that cannot be voluntarily expelled. This remainder is called *residual volume* (RV). The combination of ERV and RV is called *functional residual capacity* (FRC). This volume of residual air is believed to play a buffering role for blood oxygen and carbon dioxide saturation levels, preventing extreme fluctuation. At the end of comfortable inspiration, there is still room for more air to be inhaled; this is called *inspiratory reserve volume* (IRV). As one exercises and increases the need for oxygen, tidal volume increases, reducing both ERV and IRV. The combination of ERV and IRV plus tidal volume is called *vital capacity* (VC), which is a laboratory measurement of the maximum amount of air that can be inhaled and subsequently exhaled. These relationships are graphically demonstrated in Figure 2-7. VC varies widely by stature, gender, and the individual. A low VC per body mass reduces the amount of oxygen potentially available for metabolism, whereas a large VC-to–body mass ratio increases aerobic potential.

FRC reduces to about 54% of the normal value with immersion to the xiphoid [26]. Most of this loss is due to reduction in ERV, which decreases by 75% at this level of immersion [27]. The change in this volume may be perceived readily at poolside: While sitting on the edge of the pool exhale normally, and then expel the rest of the reserve volume forcibly. Enter the water to neck level, and perform the same experiment; the difference is highly perceptible. Little air remains to exhale at the endpoint of relaxed exhalation. ERV is reduced to 11% of VC, equal to breathing at a negative pressure of –20.5 cm of water [22]. There is some loss of RV, which drops by 15% [23]. VC decreases about 6–9% when comparing immersion to the neck to controls submerged to the xiphoid [22,23]. About 50–60% of this VC reduction is due to increased thoracic blood volume, and 40–50% is due to hydrostatic forces counteracting the inspiratory musculature [22,23]. Pressure on the rib cage shrinks the rib cage circumference by approximately 10% during submersion [22]. VC does appear to fluctuate somewhat with temperature, decreasing with cooler water immer-

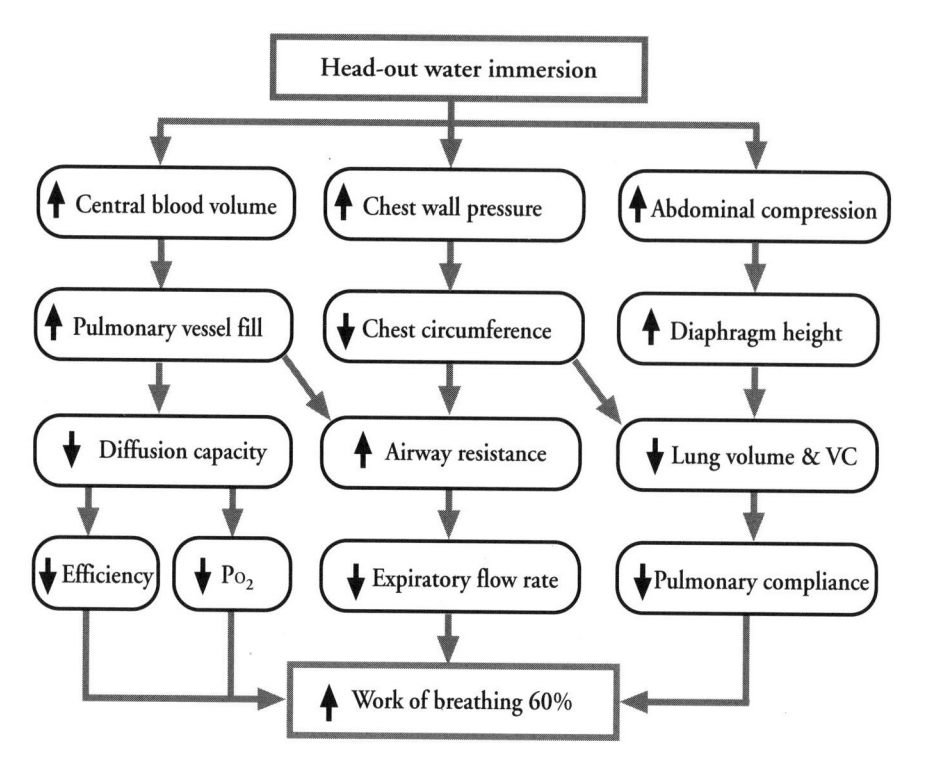

Figure 2-8. Schematic of immersion effects on respiration. (VC = vital capacity; P_{O_2} = partial pressure of oxygen.)

sion (25°C) and increasing slightly in warm water immersion (40°C) [28]. Figure 2-8 depicts the changes in pulmonary function during immersion.

The ability of the alveolar membrane to exchange gases is called *diffusion capacity*. Diffusion capacity of the lungs is reduced slightly during immersion to the neck, as is blood oxygen concentration as the lung beds become distended with blood shifted from the extremities and abdomen. Total intrapulmonary pressure shifts to the right by 16 cm of water [23], which causes airway resistance to the movement of air to increase by 58% or more because of reduced lung volume [22]. Expiratory flow rates are reduced, increasing the time needed to move air in and out of the lungs. Chest wall compliance is reduced due to the pressure of water on the chest wall, increasing pleural pressure to from −1 to +1 mm Hg [5].

The combined effect of all these changes is to increase the total work of breathing when submerged to the neck (Figure 2-9). The total work of breathing for a tidal volume of 1 liter increases by 60% during submersion to the neck. Of this increased effort three-fourths is attributable to an increase in elastic work (redistribution of blood from the thorax) and the rest to dynamic work (hydrostatic force on the thorax) [23]. Thus, for an athlete used to land-based conditioning exercises, a program of water-based exercise results in a significant workload challenge to the respiratory apparatus. This challenge can raise the efficiency of the respiratory system if the time spent in water conditioning is sufficient to achieve respiratory apparatus strength gains.

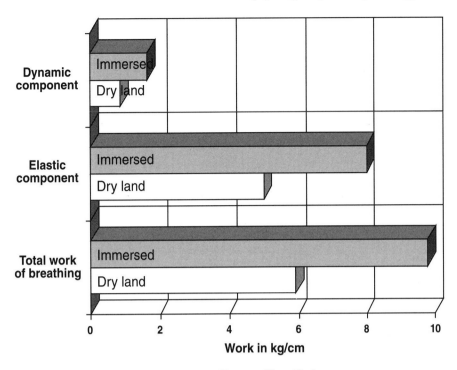

Figure 2-9. Work of breathing (energy costs of immersed breathing).

Musculoskeletal System

Water immersion causes significant effects on the musculoskeletal system as well. The effects are caused by the compressive effects of immersion as well as reflex regulation of blood vessel tone. Several of the studies previously quoted have concluded that during immersion, it is likely that most of the increased cardiac output is redistributed to skin and muscle rather than to the splanchnic beds [29]. Resting muscle blood flow has been found to increase from a dry baseline of 1.8 ml/min/100 g tissue to 4.1 ml/min/100 g tissue with immersion to the neck [30]. In the same study, xenon clearance in the tibialis anterior, a measure of tissue perfusion, during immersion to heart level was found to increase 130% above dry land clearance, essentially an identical rise to the cardiac output during immersion. Thus, oxygen delivery is significantly increased during immersion, as is the removal of muscle metabolic waste products. To resist blood pooling in dry conditions, sympathetic vasoconstriction tightens the resistance vessels of skeletal muscle. Immersion pressure removes the biological need for vasoconstriction, thus increasing muscle blood flow. Hydrostatic forces add an additional circulatory drive. Because 0.5-in. water depth produces pressure of 1 mm Hg, immersion to only 36 in. of depth results in pressure that exceeds average diastolic pressure and acts to drive out edema, muscle lactate, and other metabolic end products.

Conditioning Effects

Controversy has existed regarding the utility of a program of water-based exercise in maintaining fitness in athletes who must be sheltered from gravity during an injury recovery. For maintenance of cardiorespiratory conditioning in highly fit individuals, water running equals dry land running in its effect on maintenance of maximum $\dot{V}O_2$ when training intensities and frequencies are matched [31]. Similarly, when aquatic exercise is compared with land-based equivalent exercise in effect on maximum $\dot{V}O_2$ gains in unfit individuals, aquatic exercise is seen to achieve equivalent results, and when water temperature is low, the gains achieved are accompanied by a lower heart rate [32]. Lactate threshold more closely correlates to training performance than heart rate or $\dot{V}O_2$. Blood lactate has been found to shift to the left in relationship to oxygen uptake in both submaximal and maximal water running when compared to dry-land treadmill running [33]. Thus, water-based exercise programs may be used effectively to sustain or increase aerobic conditioning in athletes who need to keep weight off a joint, such as when in injury recovery or when in an intensive training program in which joint or bone microtrauma might occur. A key question frequently raised is whether aquatic exercise programs have sufficient specificity to provide a reasonable training venue for athletes in this situation. Hamer and Morton [34] addressed this question and found that water-based running programs did achieve significant reductions in submaximal heart rates and improved performance on graded exercise tests when compared to nonexercising controls.

Open vs. Closed Kinetic Chain Issues

An aquatic exercise program may be designed to vary the amount of gravity loading by using buoyancy as a counterforce. A joint that is moving against fixed resistance, such as the ground, forms a closed kinetic chain. Rehabilitative programs for specific joints may be more effective as either closed or open kinetic chain programs. Generally, where a normally gravity-loaded joint has undergone extensive reconstruction, many rehabilitationists feel that closed chain exercises are preferable.

Shallow-water vertical exercises generally approximate closed chain exercise, albeit with reduced joint loading because of the counterforce produced by buoyancy. Deep water exercises more generally approximate an open chain system, as do horizontal exercises, such as swimming. Paddles and other resistive equipment tend to close the kinetic chain. Aquatic programs, however, offer the ability to damp the force of movement instantaneously because of the viscous properties of water.

The effects of buoyancy and water resistance make possible high levels of energy expenditure with relatively little movement and strain on lower extremity joints [35]. Off-loading of body weight occurs as a function of immersion, but the water depth chosen may be adjusted for the amount of loading desired [35]. The amount of weight off-loading occurring through progressive immersion is shown in Figure 2-10. The spine is especially well protected during aquatic exercise programs, which facilitates early rehabilitation from back injuries.

The force exerted against the floor by the walking body is counteracted by the ground. This force is termed ground reaction force and may easily be measured through a force plate. It has been found to differ from walking on ground substantially during walking in chest-deep water [36]. Figure 2-11 shows the force plate tracing of the pressure during a gait cycle on dry land compared with chest-deep

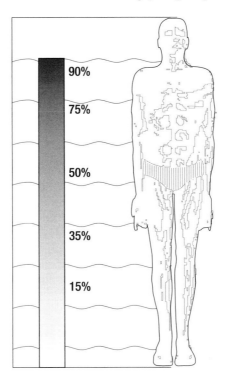

Figure 2-10. Percentage of body weight off-loaded with increasing immersion depth.

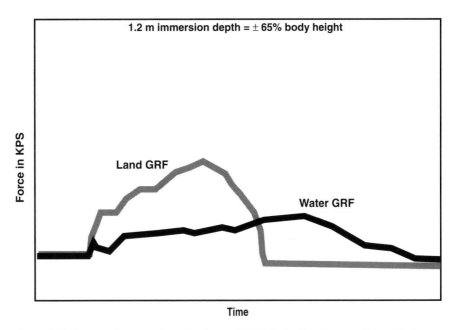

Figure 2-11. Comparative ground reaction forces (GRFs) for land and water walking. (KPS = kilopond-seconds.) (Adapted from K Nakazawa, H Yano, M Miyashita. Ground Reaction Forces During Walking in Water. In M Miyashita, Y Mutoh, AB Richardson et al. [eds], Medicine and Science in Aquatic Sports/10th FINA World Sport Medicine Congress, Medicine and Sport Science Vol 39. Basel, Switzerland: Karger AG, 1994;28.)

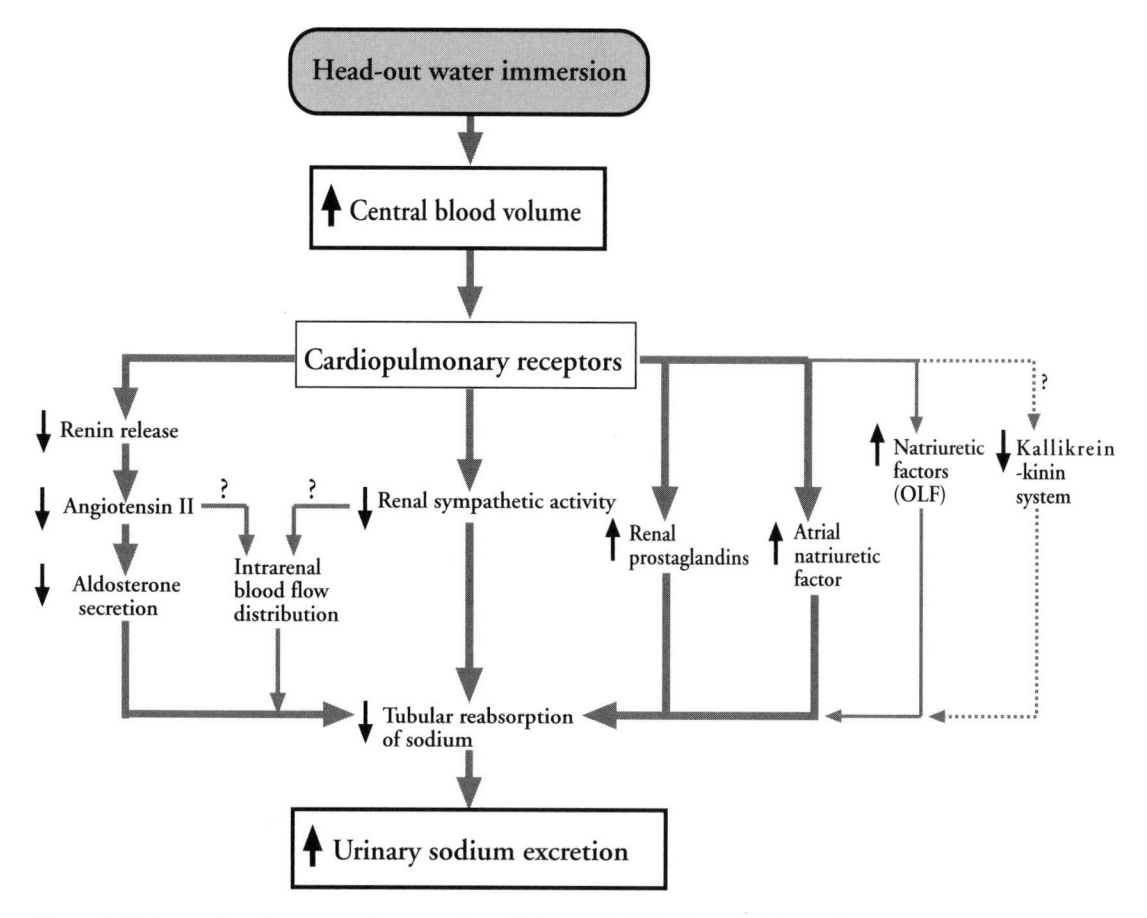

Figure 2-12. Immersion effects on sodium excretion. (OLF = ouabainlike factor.) (Adapted from M Epstein. Renal effects of head out immersion in humans: a 15-year update. Physiol Rev 1992;72:577.)

immersion. The forces generated are reduced in magnitude by more than 50%, are generated more slowly, and are transmitted over a longer time interval during water walking. Clinically, this means that less joint compression is produced and impact strain is diminished.

Renal and Endocrine Systems

Aquatic immersion has many effects on renal blood flow, on the renal regulatory systems, and on the endocrine systems (Figure 2-12). These effects have been extensively studied. Murray Epstein, one of the most skilled and prolific researchers of immersion effects on humans, published an exhaustive summary of these effects in 1992 [29]. The flow of blood to the kidneys increases immediately on immersion. This causes an increase in creatinine clearance (a measure of renal efficiency) initially on immersion [18]. Renal sympathetic nerve activity decreases due to the vagal response caused by left atrial distention, and this decrease in sympathetic nerve activity increases renal tubular sodium transport [18]. Calculated renal vascular resistance decreases by about one-third [16]. Renal venous pressure increases

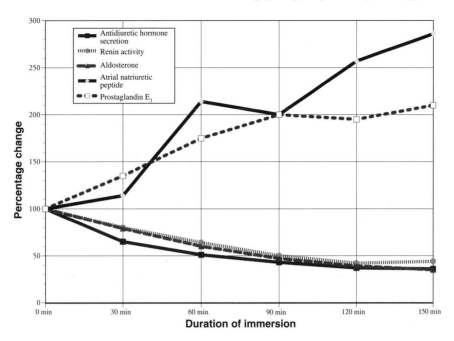

Figure 2-13. Renal hormone changes during immersion.

almost twofold [16]. Sodium excretion increases tenfold in individuals with normal total-body sodium, and this sodium excretion is accompanied by free water, creating part of the diuretic effect of immersion. This increase in sodium excretion is a time-dependent phenomenon. Sodium excretion also increases as a function of depth, due to the shifting of circulating central blood volume [14]. Release of a humeral natriuretic factor occurs through distention of the atria, and the peptide produced, atrial natriuretic peptide (ANP), facilitates sodium excretion and diuresis. ANP relaxes vascular smooth muscle and inhibits production of aldosterone; it also appears to persist for a period of time following immersion. Potassium excretion also increases with immersion [37].

Renal function is largely regulated by the hormones renin, aldosterone, and antidiuretic hormone (ADH). All these hormones are greatly affected by immersion (Figure 2-13). Aldosterone controls sodium reabsorption in the distal renal tubule and accounts for most of the sodium loss with immersion. Suppression begins on immersion, reaches maximum at 2 hours, but falls to 60% of maximum at 3 hours of immersion time. Aldosterone production is reduced to 80% of control at 30 minutes of immersion time, 60% of control at 1 hour, and maximizes at 35% of control at 3 hours. ADH release is suppressed with immersion by 50% or more, which is the other major contributor to diuresis [15,29]. Another factor important in sodium regulation is ANP. ANP reduces the reabsorption of sodium in the distal renal tubular system, thus increasing urinary sodium content. Immersion produces a prompt and continuing increase in ANP [34]. Renal prostaglandin E secretion increases steadily through the first 2 hours of immersion and then drops gently over the next 3 hours [29]. Renin stimulates angiotensin, which in turn stimulates aldosterone release. Renin activity reduces by 20% of control at 30 minutes of immersion, 38% at 1 hour,

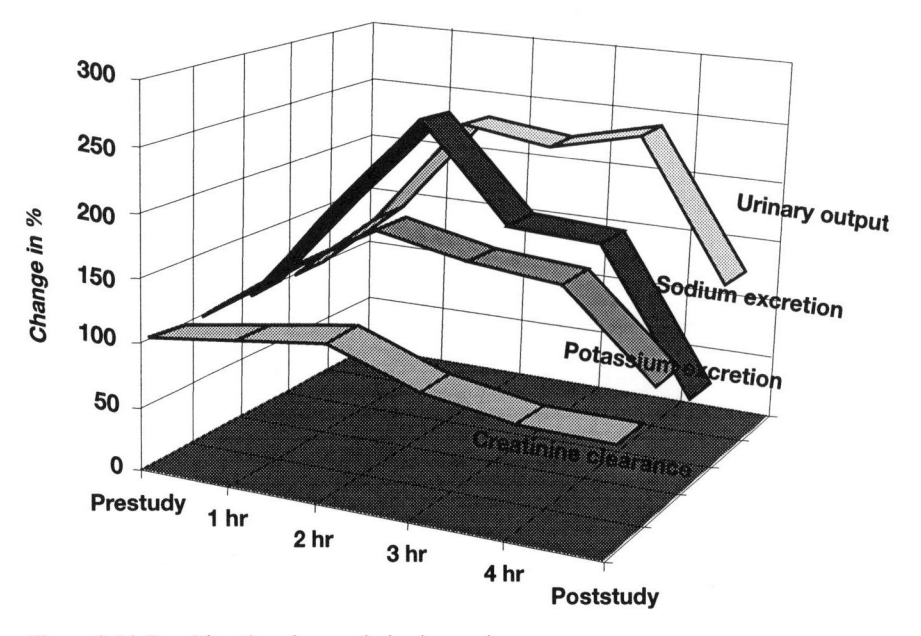

Figure 2-14. Renal function changes during immersion.

and maximizes at 62% of control at 3 hours of immersion. Plasma renin activity is reduced by 33–50% at 2 hours of immersion to the neck [14].

Overall, immersion-induced central volume expansion causes increased urinary output accompanied by significant sodium and potassium excretion, beginning almost immediately on immersion, steadily increasing through several hours of immersion, and gently tapering off over subsequent hours. Figure 2-14 shows these time-dependent changes in urinary excretion.

The combined effect of the renal responses, the autonomic responses, and the cardiovascular responses on blood pressure has been studied intensively, with varying results. During sustained immersion in neutral-temperature water, blood pressure does not appear to change greatly. During neutral-temperature immersion, patients with essential hypertension often show lowered blood pressure [20]. These combined renal and sympathetic nervous system effects typically lower blood pressure in the immersed hypertensive individual during sustained immersion and create a period of lowered pressure for a period of hours thereafter.

Accompanying the renal hormone effects are changes in the autonomic nervous system neurotransmitters, called *catecholamines*, which act to regulate vascular resistance, cardiac rate, and cardiac force. The most important of these are epinephrine, norepinephrine, and dopamine. Catecholamine levels begin changing immediately on immersion (Figure 2-15) [38,39].

Central and Peripheral Nervous Systems

Many effects have been observed anecdotally throughout centuries of aquatic environment use for health maintenance and restoration but they are difficult to study. Predominant among these are the relaxation effect of water immersion and the effect

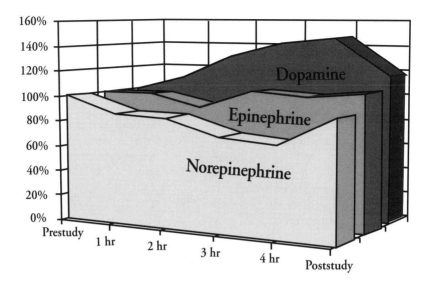

Figure 2-15. Catecholamine responses to immersion.

that water immersion has on pain perception. Skin sensor nerve endings are affected, including temperature, touch, and pressure receptors. Sensory overflow has been suggested to be the mechanism by which pain is less well perceived when the affected body part is immersed in water. Pain modulation is consequently affected with a rise in pain threshold, which increases with temperature and water turbulence, producing the known therapeutic effect of agitated whirlpool immersion.

A relaxation effect is produced by a central process that is not understood, is likely multifactorial, and is likely produced within the reticular activating system deep within the brain. Mood state has been found to improve following dry land exercise but has not been studied in an aquatic environment. Similarly, both anxiety and depression are reduced following dry land exercise, and research to test these effects following aquatic exercise has not been done. Plasma catecholamines are known to increase during exercise and decrease following exercise; the rise decreases with training effect, which may account for some of these psychological changes [40].

Weight Control Issues

Water exercise seems to have a fat-sparing quality because similar exercise intensities and durations do not produce similar body fat decreases [41,42]. It has been noted that elite aquatic distance athletes do not lower their body fat percentages to the same extent that elite track distance athletes do, corroborating this research. Nonetheless, aquatic exercise programs may be highly beneficial in the restoration of fitness in obese patients because of the protective effects against heavy joint loading achieved in the aquatic environment. The ability to achieve an aerobic exercise level for sufficient time to produce a conditioning effect may be difficult in this population on dry land, and a program that begins in water and moves to land as tolerance builds may be the most effective method of achieving both conditioning and weight loss.

CONCLUSION

As the information in this chapter demonstrates, immersing the body in water produces many physiologic effects, which have been subjectively reported since nearly the beginning of recorded history, and the effects have been therapeutically used over centuries of medical history. Recent research has contributed to the understanding of the physiologic changes that create these therapeutic effects. There are, however, many areas that merit more study.

The cardiac effects produced by immersion are profound and salutary, both for the healthy heart and usually for the rehabilitating heart. Through an understanding of the effects of the aquatic environment on cardiac workload, a program of progressive cardiac strengthening may be developed, so that even severely deconditioned or injured hearts may functionally improve.

Equally important are the effects of immersion on the pulmonary system. Because the respiratory apparatus must work harder when immersed, respiratory muscle strengthening occurs, and the processes of respiration may be enhanced. A program of regular aquatic exercise should produce a significant training effect that is objectively and subjectively apparent. This effect has been studied in humans with spinal injuries and clearly does occur [43,44]. It also happens in asthma-afflicted individuals, as is discussed in Chapter 7.

The effects on the circulatory and autonomic nervous systems facilitate improvement in muscle blood flow and an increase in rate of removal of metabolic waste and injury products from deep within muscle tissues. Consequently, both normal exercising muscle and healing muscle and ligament structures experience beneficial effects.

The effects of immersion on the renal system include promoting the excretion of metabolic waste products; assisting the regulation of sodium, potassium, and water; and generally lowering blood pressure. The renal effects persist longer than the period of immersion, often lasting many hours or even days.

All of the above-mentioned effects are therapeutically useful. That these effects can occur in an environment that is clinically safe, promotes the reduction of pain, and is even pleasurable is unique. Aquatic rehabilitation is vastly underused. We have been lured by the appeal of high technology and advanced pharmacology, often at the cost of greater medical expense and side-effect complications. A return to the roots of rehabilitation is appropriate.

All these effects are good reasons to use the aquatic environment in training and rehabilitation. Yet much research opportunity exists for further documenting the mechanisms producing the effects and studying the most efficient means of achieving desired results in conditioning and therapy. In particular, research is needed on fat metabolism and water exercise, bone and calcium metabolism as a function of aquatic exercise, and hypertension management through aquatic exercise.

Aquatic facilities are widely available, and public acceptance is already high, so there are tremendous potential public health benefits to be achieved through programs targeted at the most significant physiologic consequences of aging: hypertension, cardiovascular disease, arthritis and other joint pathology, and obesity and deconditioning. There are sound physiologic reasons for speculation that a broader public participation in aquatic programs could lower our national health care budget while preserving improved function for the general population. Aquatic programs for achieving fitness and restoring function may be designed for a broad range of individuals through an understanding of the fundamental principles of aquatic physics and the application of those principles to human physiology.

REFERENCES

1. Kuroda PK. What Is Water? In S Licht (ed), Medical Hydrology. Baltimore: Waverly, 1963;1.
2. Giancoli DC. Fluids. In Physics—Principles with Applications (2nd ed). Englewood Cliffs, NJ: Prentice-Hall, 1985;184.
3. Bloomfield J, Fricker P, Fitch K. Textbook of Science and Medicine in Sport. Champaign, IL: Human Kinetics Books, 1992;5.
4. Somers L. Diving Physics. In AA Bove, JC Davis (eds), Diving Medicine (2nd ed). Philadelphia: Saunders, 1990;9.
5. Arborelius M, Balldin UI, Lilja B, Lundgren CE. Hemodynamic changes in man during immersion with the head above water. Aerospace Med 1972;43:593.
6. Risch WD, Koubenec HJ, Beckmann U, et al. The effect of graded immersion on heart volume, central venous pressure, pulmonary blood distribution and heart rate in man. Pflügers Arch 1978;374:117.
7. Weston CFM, O'Hare JP, Evans JM, Corrall RJM. Haemodynamic changes in man during immersion in water at different temperatures. Clin Sci (Colch) 1987;73:613.
8. Schlant RC, Sonnenblick EH. Normal Physiology of the Cardiovascular System. In JW Hurst (ed), The Heart (6th ed). New York: McGraw-Hill, 1986;51.
9. McArdle WD, Katch FI, Katch VL. Exercise Physiology, Energy, Nutrition and Human Performance (3rd ed). Malvern, PA: Lea & Febiger, 1991;435.
10. Haffor AA, Mohler JG, Harrison AC. Effects of water immersion on cardiac output of lean and fat male subjects at rest and during exercise. Aviat Space Environ Med 1991;62:125.
11. Evans BW, Cureton KJ, Purvis JW. Metabolic and circulatory responses to walking and jogging in water. Res Q 1978;49:442.
12. Dressendorfer RH, Morlock JF, Baker DG, Hong SK. Effects of head-out water immersion on cardiorespiratory responses to maximal cycling exercise. Undersea Biomedical Research 1976;3:183.
13. McMurray RG, Fieselman CC, Avery KE, Sheps DS. Exercise hemodynamics in water and on land in patients with coronary artery disease. Cardiopulmonary Rehabil 1988;8:69.
14. Tanaka N, Tei C. Hydrothermal effects in congestive heart disease. Circulation 1994 (in press).
15. Tajima F, Sagawa S, Iwamoto J, et al. Renal and endocrine responses in the elderly during head-out immersion. Am J Physiol 1988;254:R977. (Regulatory Integrative Comp. Physiol. 23)
16. Weston CFM, O'Hare JP, Evans JM, Corrall RJM. Haemodynamic changes in man during immersion in water at different temperatures. Clin Sci (Colch) 1987;73:613.
17. Claybaugh JR, Pendergast DR, Davis JE, et al. Fluid conservation in athletic responses to water intake, supine posture, and immersion. J Appl Physiol 1986;61:7.
18. Epstein M. Cardiovascular and renal effects of head-out water immersion in man. Circ Res 1976;39:620.
19. Coruzzi PAA, Novarini A, Biggi A, et al. Low pressure receptor activity and exaggerated naturiesis in essential hypertension. Nephron 1985;40:309.
20. Gleim GW, Nicholas JA. Metabolic costs and heart rate responses to treadmill walking in water at different depths and temperatures. Am J Sports Med 1989;17:248.
21. Borg GAV. Perceived exertion as an indicator of somatic stress. Scand J Rehabil Med 1970;2:92.
22. Glass RA. Comparative biomechanical and physiological responses of suspended deep water running to hard surface running [unpublished thesis]. Auburn, AL: Auburn University, 1987, PE (3039f).
23. Borg GAV. Psychophysical bases of perceived exertion. Med Sci Sports Exerc 1992;14:377.

24. Bishop PA, Frazier S, Smith J, Jacobs D. Physiological responses to treadmill and water running. Phys Sports Med 1989;17:87.

25. Wilder R, Brennan D. Physiological responses to deep water running in athletes. Sports Med 1993;16:374.

26. Agostoni E, Gurtner G, Torri G, Rahn H. Respiratory mechanics during submersion and negative pressure breathing. J Appl Physiol 1966;21:253.

27. Hong SK, Cerretelli P, Cruz JC, Rahn H. Mechanics of respiration during submersion in water. J Appl Physiol 1969;27:535.

28. Choukroun ML, Varene P. Adjustments in oxygen transport during head-out immersion in water at various temperatures. J Appl Physiol 1990;68:1475.

29. Epstein M. Renal effects of head out immersion in humans: a 15-year update. Physiol Rev 1992;72:563.

30. Balldin UI, Lundgren CEG, Lundvall J, Mellander S. Changes in the elimination of 133xenon from the anterior tibial muscle in man induced by immersion in water and by shifts in body position. Aerospace Medicine 1971;42:489.

31. Gatti CJ, Young RJ, Glad HL. Effect of water-training in the maintenance of cardiorespiratory endurance of athletes. Br J Sports Med 1979;13:162.

32. Avellini BA, Shapiro Y, Pandolf KB. Cardio-respiratory physical training in water and on land. Eur J Appl Physiol 1983;50:255.

33. Svedenhag J, Seger J. Running on land and in water: comparative exercise physiology. Med Sci Sports Exerc 1992;24:1158.

34. Hamer TW, Morton AR. Water-running: training effects and specificity of aerobic, anaerobic and muscular parameters following an eight-week interval training programme. Aust J Sci Med Sport 1990;22:13.

35. Harrison RA, Hillman M, Bulstrode S. Loading of the lower limb when walking partially immersed. Physiotherapy 1992;78:165.

36. Nakazawa K, Yano H, Miyashita M. Ground Reaction Forces During Walking in Water. In M Miyashita, Y Mutoh, AB Richardson (eds), Medicine and Science in Aquatic Sports. 10th FINA World Sport Medicine Congress, Medicine and Sport Science, Vol 39. Basel, Switzerland: Karger AG, 1994;28.

37. Epstein M, Lifschitz D, Hoffman D, Stein J. Relationship between renal prostaglandin E and renal sodium handling during water immersion in normal man. Circ Res 1979;45:71.

38. Grossman E, Goldstein DS, Hoffman A, et al. Effects of water immersion on sympathoadrenal and dopa-dopamine systems in humans. Am J Physiol 1992;262:R993. (Regulatory Integrative Comp. Physiol. 31)

39. Krishna D, Sowers J. Catecholamine responses to central volume expansion produced by head-out water immersion and saline infusion. J Clin Endocrinol Metab 1983;56:998.

40. Connelly TP, Sheldahl LM, Tristani FE, et al. Effect of increased central blood volume with water immersion on plasma catecholamines during exercise. J Appl Physiol 1990;69:651.

41. Gwinup G. Weight loss without dietary restriction: efficacy of different forms of aerobic exercise. Am J Sports Med 1987;15:275.

42. Kieres J, Plowman S. Effects of swimming and land exercises on body composition of college students. J Sports Med Phys Fitness 1991;31:192.

43. Pachalski A, Mekarski T. Effect of swimming on increasing of cardiorespiratory capacity in paraplegics. Paraplegia 1980;18:190.

44. Tajima F, Sagawa J, Iwamoto J, et al. Cardiovascular, renal, and endocrine responses in male quadriplegics during head-out immersion. Am J Physiol 1990; 258:R1424. (Regulatory Integrative Comp. Physiol. 27)

3

Aquatic Rehabilitation for the Treatment of Neurologic Disorders

David M. Morris

Patients with neurologic disorders have complex impairments, which may contribute to problems with walking, transferring, and reaching. Aquatic rehabilitation offers a unique, versatile approach to the treatment of these impairments and the disabilities they create.

The need for neurorehabilitation strategies has increased in recent years. Improved technology and medical management have allowed more individuals to survive head injuries, brain tumors, strokes, birth injuries, and premature birth [1,2]. In addition, longer life expectancies may account for the increased prevalence of neurologic disorders. Currently, our health care system requires increased accountability by the rehabilitation professional, especially with regard to reimbursement for services. Therefore, neurorehabilitation professionals must seek ever more effective treatment strategies. Aquatic rehabilitation has been advocated by many as a useful treatment modality for patients with neurologic disorders [3–10]. The unique properties of water, particularly buoyancy and turbulence, enable the design of effective and versatile treatment programs [3–6]. Specific benefits of the aquatic environment include weight relief and ease of movement. These characteristics allow movement exploration, strengthening, and functional activity training, often before patients can perform the same on land. Also, the supportive properties of water allow easy handling of patients by aquatic therapy professionals. This chapter examines the problems encountered by patients with neurologic disorders, general principles guiding neurotreatment, and aquatic neurorehabilitation approaches. For the purposes of this chapter, neurologic diagnoses include stroke, head injury, spinal cord injury, cerebral palsy, brain tumors, and Parkinson's disease.

DESCRIPTION OF NEUROLOGIC DISORDERS

Problems encountered during the treatment of neurologic disorders can be classified according to the International Classification of Impairments, Disabilities, and Handicaps (ICIDH) [11]. According to the ICIDH, an *impairment* is any loss or abnormality of an organ, structure, or function. A *disability* is any reduction, partial or total, in the capacity to carry out any functional activity within the range considered normal for the average human being. Typical disabilities include walking, transferring, and reaching. A *handicap* is an externally imposed disadvantage that limits or prevents the fulfillment of usual social roles, depending on age, gender, and culture. Typical neurologic handicaps include physical barriers, attitudinal barriers, lowered expectations (the patient's), and fear (the patient's). The application of aquatic rehabilitation approaches can influence neurologic disorders at any or all of these levels.

REHABILITATION OF PATIENTS WITH NEUROLOGIC DISORDERS

Several major changes have occurred in the rehabilitation of neurologic disorders. These changes, occurring in response to societal and technologic advances, have been outlined by Gordon and Horak [1,2].

Motor Control Models

Assumptions about how humans create and control movement profoundly influence the way patients are evaluated and treated. Three motor control models—the reflex model, the hierarchic model, and the systems model—have received the most attention from the medical community [1,2]. The reflex model assumes that human movement occurs in response to sensory input to the central nervous system (CNS). For example, when a person is sitting in a car that quickly accelerates, sensory input into the vestibular system facilitates forward neck and trunk flexion and protective extension of the arms. These movements counterbalance backward displacement and prevent the individual from falling back into the car seat. In studies with animals whose sensory endings were intentionally destroyed, the animals still exhibited coordinated, purposeful movement [12] as well as the ability to move in anticipation of a postural disturbance (feed-forward control) [13]. Therefore, a reflex model does not fully explain the production of skilled movement.

The hierarchic model views the CNS as a top-down control pattern in which the higher centers of the cerebral cortex control the lower centers of the brain stem and spinal cord. The lower centers are in charge of more primitive, reflex types of movement; the higher centers control the more complex, voluntary types of movement. Limitations of this model have been cited based on studies in which experimentally induced lesions of the midbrains of cats (i.e., disruption of connections between higher and lower CNS structures) failed to prohibit coordinated, purposeful movement [14]. Reflexive movements may appropriately over-ride voluntary movements for functional purposes in normal humans. For example, when stepping on a nail, the injured foot reflexively withdraws while the supporting limb extends [2]. A purely hierarchic view of motor control appears inaccurate.

Unlike the reflex and hierarchic models, the systems model does not regard the CNS as solely responsible for motor control. In this model, movement results from interaction among many different kinds of systems, including environmental, musculoskeletal, and sensorimotor. No particular system is always in control of others;

instead, each may be more important depending on the task at hand. In addition, the system cannot be explained by exploring each system separately. In other words, resulting movements occur secondary to interactions between the systems. There are problems with this view of motor control. The underlying systems whose interactions result in movement have yet to be well defined, and the relationship of these systems to neuroanatomic structures is not well understood [2].

Neurorehabilitation Models

The treatment approaches used by rehabilitation professionals are many and varied. Most, however, can be easily aligned with one of three models of neurorehabilitation [1,2]. In the early days of physical rehabilitation, most patients served by therapists had poliomyelitis. The prevalent rehabilitation model was a muscle re-education model wherein therapists strengthened weak musculature and provided orthopedic support or bracing for body segments to which strength would not return. Patients with neurologic disorders were treated in an identical manner. Many professionals were dissatisfied with the muscle re-education approach. The plasticity (ability to recover) of the CNS was not considered, and patients with neurologic disorders often had more difficulty with patterns of movement and could not isolate specific muscle actions. This led to a general shift to a neurotherapeutic facilitation approach.

Developed in the 1950s, the neurotherapeutic facilitation model was the basic philosophy followed by many theorists, including the Bobaths, Knott and Voss, Ayres, Rood, and Stockmeyer. Treatment approaches developed from this model dominated the field of neurorehabilitation for the next 30 years and still have a strong influence on rehabilitation practices. With this model, therapists facilitate normal (or desirable) movement patterns by providing sensory input. Careful steps are taken to inhibit abnormal muscle tone and to avoid abnormal movement patterns and primitive reflexes.

Dissatisfaction with this model arises from the apparent lack of functional carryover; that is, the avoidance of primitive or abnormal movement patterns did not necessarily produce normal functional movement. Also, the patient's role was largely passive, responding to the therapist's sensory input. Finally, the model explained neurologic movement disorders as the result of an aberrant CNS; it failed to take into account musculoskeletal and environmental influences on movement.

In recent years, another major shift has occurred. Research of contemporary movement science indicates that functionally oriented neurotreatment, in which patients are more active problem solvers, may be more effective than treatments based on earlier models. This has led many rehabilitation experts to endorse a task-oriented approach to neurorehabilitation. Strategies based on this school of thought incorporate the practice of specific functional goals. Patients learn to develop effective, efficient compensatory strategies to carry out tasks. They also learn adaptability to performing these tasks under a variety of musculoskeletal and environmental constraints (e.g., on different surfaces, with different obstacles to avoid, in different lighting). More attention is placed on the patient's ability to perform a task than on which specific movement pattern is used. Like the other neurorehabilitation models, a task-oriented model has dissatisfying aspects. Many patients receiving neurotreatment have a limited ability to participate as active problem solvers due to major physical or mental impairments. Also, it is difficult to retrain the ability to anticipate the need for a particular motor strategy.

In review:

1. The muscle re-education model does not consider incorporating researched motor control.
2. The neurotherapeutic facilitation model assumes reflex and hierarchic principles of motor control.
3. The task-oriented approach incorporates principles from all three models of motor control.

Therefore, more contemporary models of neurorehabilitation must incorporate an expanded view of the mechanisms of movement.

AQUATIC NEUROREHABILITATION

Several aquatic rehabilitation approaches have been promoted for treating patients with neurologic disorders. The guiding principles of each and their relation to general neurorehabilitation approaches is described here.

General Guidelines for Treatment Design

A number of factors must be considered when designing aquatic rehabilitation programs. In the author's opinion, the following factors are most influential in aquatic treatment design for neurologically impaired patients [12,13].

Depth of the Water

Because buoyant support increases as more of the body is submerged, patients who have difficulty standing can perform exercises more easily in deeper water. Therefore, exercises should be performed first in deeper water with a progression to more shallow depths. One exception to this guideline is arm exercises. Performing such activities in shallow water may prevent patients from submerging the entire upper extremity to maximize buoyancy assistance to movement or resistance from the water's drag.

Unilateral vs. Bilateral Movements

The resistant drag produced with movement in the water increases effort for the patient. When a submerged extremity is moved, the increased effort challenges the stability provided by the moving individual's trunk and proximal segments. This increased effort can be minimized if the patient moves only one extremity, particularly if the other extremity is used to provide additional stability (e.g., holding on to the side of the pool, standing on the pool's floor). As the patient's ability to stabilize improves, bilateral movements should be attempted. Regarding resistive force produced and challenging proximal stability, asymmetric bilateral movements (e.g., moving the right shoulder into flexion while simultaneously moving the left shoulder into extension) are generally easier than symmetric bilateral movements (e.g., both shoulders moving into flexion simultaneously).

Distal Stabilization

When the distal end of a moving body segment is contacting an object with stable properties, the patient performing the activity can incorporate the support into his or her ability to stabilize. Therefore, these distal end–stable activities are generally easier to accomplish than when the distal end of a moving body segment moves free of stabilization (distal end free). Stability-providing objects may or may not be fixed and stationary. For example, although a free-floating buoyant ring is not fixed to the side of the pool, it still provides stability. Examples of distal end–stable aquatic activities include resting a hand on a kickboard and moving across the surface of the water in shoulder-horizontal abduction-adduction or performing most Bad Ragaz ring method (BRRM) activities. Distal end–free aquatic activities are performed without the additional distal support from an external source. Examples of these activities include performing a swimming stroke or deep-water running.

Speed and Excursion of Movement

As a person immersed in water slightly increases the speed of his movement, the resistance encountered dramatically increases. Similarly, as patients move through greater range of motion (ROM), the activity difficulty also increases. Therefore, patients should begin activities slowly and through small ROM and gradually increase both as skill allows. A general guideline for patients is to instruct them to move as quickly and as far as they can and still do the activity in a comfortable, correct manner. Improper movement patterns are an indication that the patient is exceeding his or her abilities of speed and excursion.

Patient's Position

As on land, certain body positions assumed in the water are easier to control than others. Unfortunately, many patients automatically assume the least stable positions when allowed to do so. Campion describes four positions commonly assumed during therapeutic pool activities: the ball, cube, triangle, and stick positions [5]. These positions are listed from the most to least stable. Although the ball position is the most stable, it is probably the least used during patient care. Instead, the cube is the most practical for use with patients. By submerging the body, assuming a sitting position, and extending the arms, the patient positions the trunk and extremities in a manner that maximizes the buoyant support provided by the water (Figure 3-1). As the patient gains more skill and independence, he or she can assume the triangle position (Figure 3-2) and the stick position (Figure 3-3), in which less of the body is submerged and supported by buoyant forces. Less-skilled patients should first attempt activities in a more stable position and move toward performing in less stable positions as skill progresses.

Water Shiatsu

Water shiatsu (WATSU) was developed by Harold Dull at Harbin Hot Springs, California [15]. Dull describes the technique as Zen shiatsu principles applied to people floating in the water. WATSU was created as a wellness technique; it was not origi-

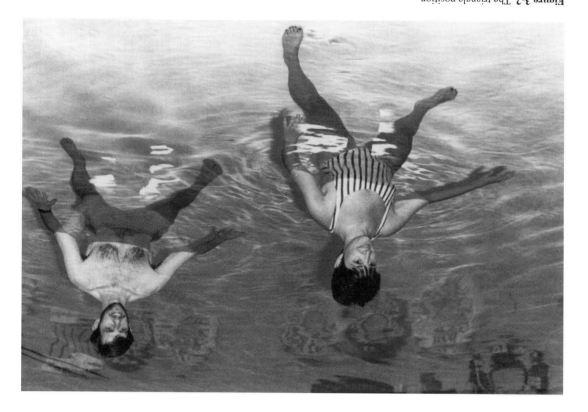

Figure 3-2. The triangle position.

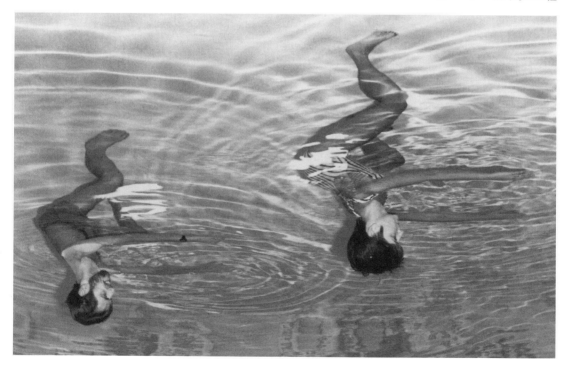

Figure 3-1. The cube position.

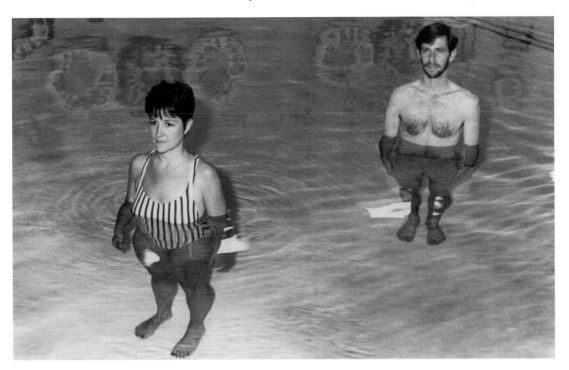

Figure 3-3. The stick position.

nally intended for patients with neurologic disorders. Rehabilitation therapists have applied the approach to patients with a variety of physical disorders, however, and anecdotal reports indicate clinical success. Based on Eastern medicine theory, WATSU stretches the body's meridians (pathways of energy). Through stretching, these pathways are thought to be brought closer to the body's surface, where energy can be released. These effects are enhanced by rotational movements that release blocked energy from joint articulations. As a completely passive recipient, the patient experiences profound relaxation from the water's support and the continual, rhythmic movement that flows gracefully from one position to the next. The stretches comprise specifically described transitions and sequences of movement. In general, the therapist stabilizes or moves one segment of the body while movement through the water, resulting in a drag effect, stretches another segment. Once the transitions and sequences are learned, therapists are encouraged to vary them according to the needs and limitations of the patient.

Water Shiatsu for Patients with
Neurologic Disorders

Patients with neurologic disorders often exhibit ROM limitations secondary to soft-tissue restrictions [16]. These limitations can negatively influence functional recovery by preventing patients from moving into positions that are biomechanically efficient. Also, many tone and voluntary movement disorders are magnified when muscle tissue becomes shortened, creating increased resistance to movement

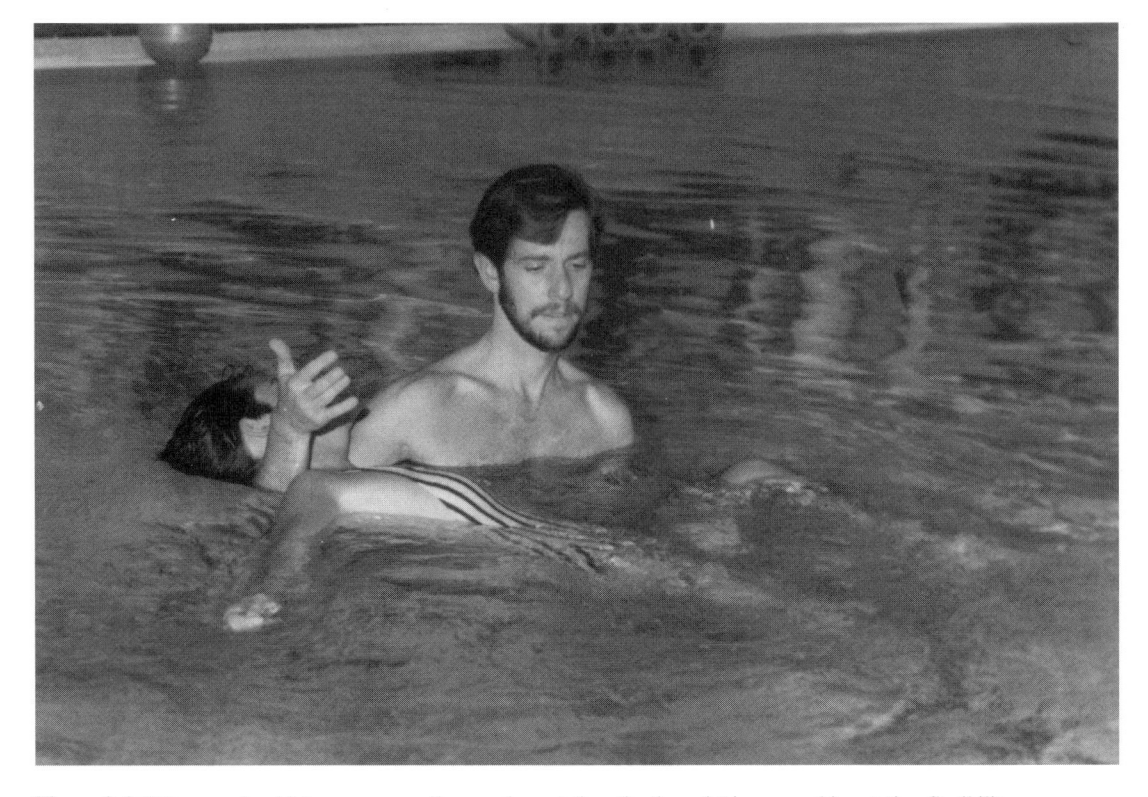

Figure 3-4. Using a water shiatsu maneuver, the near leg rotation, the therapist increases hip rotation flexibility.

[16,17]. The application of WATSU to these tight body segments can improve flexibility. This technique is particularly helpful when applied at the beginning of a treatment session, preparing the patient to move in a less restricted fashion during more active portions of the treatment session. Maneuvers that may have specific applications to patients with neurologic impairments are the near leg rotation (promoting internal and external hip rotation) (Figure 3-4), the leg push (promoting hip extension), and the accordion (promoting hip and trunk flexion) [15]. WATSU can be best described as a muscle re-education approach because specific impairments (usually tight muscles and joints) are targeted for treatment with little regard to the models of motor control.

Bad Ragaz Ring Method

The BRRM was developed in the 1930s in Bad Ragaz, Switzerland [4,18]. The technique has been modified through the years and has been dramatically influenced by proprioceptive neuromuscular facilitation (PNF), a therapeutic exercise technique used on land. BRRM is similar to PNF in that the therapist guides the patient through specific patterns of movement to increase strength and ROM. Both techniques include activities for the arms, legs, and trunk and may use unilateral or bilateral patterns. Of the bilateral patterns, some are symmetric (both sides of the body moving in the same direction) and some are asymmetric (each side moving in a different direction).

In both BRRM and PNF, the therapist gives the patient specific movement instructions (e.g., "bring your right knee to your left shoulder") and encourages a movement progression of distal to proximal segments of the body. In BRRM, the patient is floating either prone or supine in the water with flotation support at the neck, hips, and occasionally the extremities. The therapist places his or her hands on designated spots on specific segments of the patient's body while instructing the patient to move in the desired direction (Figure 3-5). The therapist thus serves as a point of stability from which the patient moves, generating resistance from the turbulent drag effects of the surrounding water. Generally, resistance to movement is encountered in every direction of movement (i.e., flexion and extension) because the body is completely surrounded by water. Unlike PNF, in which the therapist manually applies graded resistance to the patient's movements, the BRRM allows the patient to determine the amount of resistance encountered based on speed of movement. Using this method, therapists can increase the difficulty of the activity by placing their stabilizing hold more distally. Such strategies do not necessarily increase the resistance to movement but do increase the complexity of the activity because the patient must control larger segments of his or her body during the movement. Therapists are cautioned to stand in depths of water that allow them to form a stabilizing base for the patient's movements. Water depths above the therapist's eighth thoracic vertebra generally prevent the therapist from maintaining a fixed position, decreasing the effectiveness of the therapeutic application. At times, the therapist may use an overflow principle with the BRRM by stabilizing and resisting one portion of the body to encourage activity in another.

Use for Patients with Neurologic Disorders

The BRRM was designed for a variety of movement problems, mainly musculoskeletal. The technique can be effectively applied to the treatment of neurologic impairments that include voluntary movement deficit, weakness, and decreased ROM. Many patients with neurologic disorders lack the ability to stabilize multiple segments of their body, even when horizontally supported in the water. Therefore, these patients often require additional flotation support around the trunk to ensure safety and security. When working with patients exhibiting voluntary movement deficits, emphasis should be placed on smooth movement through the ROM, as opposed to quick, resistance-generating movement typically used to improve pure strength deficits.

It is common for patients with voluntary movement deficits to have difficulty relaxing muscle groups following a contraction [16,17,19]. This prevents subsequent movement from contractions in antagonistic muscle groups. The result is a rigid coactivation of muscles surrounding a joint, preventing movement in any direction. The BRRM can be modified by passively moving the patient in directions where this prolonged contraction occurs, allowing voluntary contraction of the antagonistic muscle. The therapist progressively lessens assistance through the ROM as the patient slowly gains better reciprocal inhibition control (i.e., can voluntarily relax the antagonistic group). Eventually, many patients develop the skill to move smoothly and reciprocally throughout that segment of the body. BRRM resembles a neurotherapeutic facilitation approach in that it encourages improved skill in specific patterns of movement.

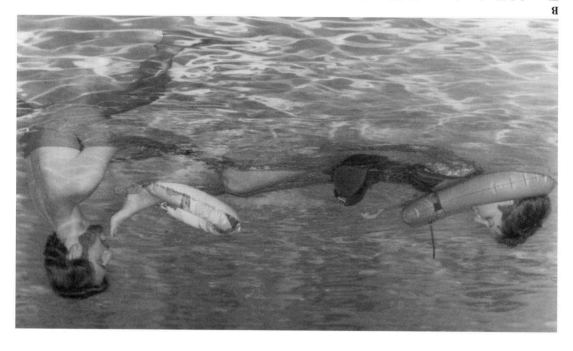

A

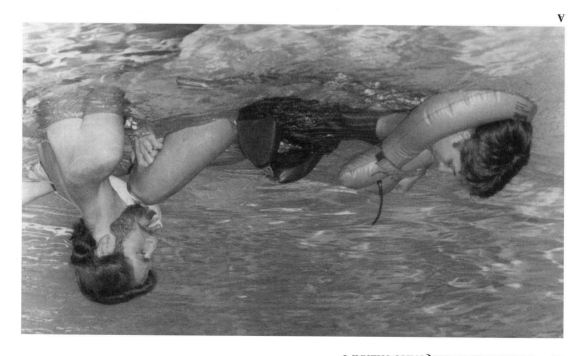

B

Figure 3-5. The therapist uses a Bad Ragaz ring method pattern to facilitate or strengthen hip flexion, knee flexion, ankle dorsiflexion, and return. A. The patient moves toward the therapist to strengthen/improve hip flexion, knee flexion, and ankle dorsiflexion. B. The patient moves away from the therapist to strengthen/improve hip extension, knee extension, and ankle plantar flexion.

Table 3-1. The 10-Point Program of the Halliwick Method

Phase 1: Adjustment to water
  1. Mental adjustment
  2. Disengagement
Phase 2: Rotation control
  3. Vertical rotation control
  4. Lateral rotation control
  5. Combined rotation control
Phase 3: Control of movement in water
  6. Use of upthrust
  7. Balance in stillness
  8. Turbulent gliding
Phase 4: Movement in water
  9. Basic progression
 10. Swimming progression

Halliwick Method

Developed by James McMillan in the 1930s at the Halliwick School for Girls in England, the Halliwick method is based on principles of hydrodynamics and human development [5,6,20,21]. The approach is intended as a swimming instruction technique, yet many of its activities and principles can be applied to specific therapeutic intervention. In general swimming instruction, each patient is assigned an individual instructor. This patient-instructor pair becomes one of a group of pairs, usually consisting of four to six pairs per group. Games are often used to teach skills and reinforce the principles of the method. In specific therapeutic intervention, however, activities are often conducted with each patient individually. The Halliwick method, best described as a neurotherapeutic facilitation rehabilitation technique, follows a disengagement principle. Therapists or instructors use activities to facilitate patterns of movement with careful consideration of the activity's level of difficulty and the amount of manual guidance provided. Specifically, the therapist starts with easy activities and guides the patient manually to ensure correct execution of the movement. As the patient becomes more skilled with the movement, the therapist reduces the amount of assistance provided (disengaging) and increases the activity's level of difficulty.

Finally, when the patient masters the activity, the therapist creates turbulence around the patient's body to challenge skill and subsequently reinforce learning. Activities are designed with consideration of general principles outlined in a 10-point program (Table 3-1). These general principles can be described as part of four phases, as follows:

Phase 1: Adjustment to Water
1. Mental adjustment. Developing the patient's comfort while in the water is stressed. This is accomplished through proper handling and educating patients regarding the effects of water on their movements. As a result, patients should never be fearful in the water.
2. Disengagement. The disengagement principle is used to plan and execute all activities. This progression is believed to best teach and reinforce skill. Activities in vertical positions (i.e., sitting, standing) are easier to accomplish than those in horizontal positions (i.e., prone, supine). Therefore, the approach uses vertical positions

earlier in skill development. Because this is the opposite of how skill is developed in a gravity environment (i.e., infants gain skill in supine before sitting and standing), the Halliwick method is said to use a reversed developmental sequence.

Phase 2: Rotation Control. Using the skills of rotation control, patients can change their position in the water. Head movements are emphasized because they greatly influence the position of the body in the water.

3. Vertical rotation control. Movements in a frontal plane are encouraged (i.e., moving from supine to upright to prone). These motions are usually controlled with neck flexion and extension.

4. Lateral rotation control. Movements in a longitudinal plane are encouraged (i.e., rolling from supine to prone). These movements are usually controlled with neck rotation.

5. Combined rotation control. A corkscrew-like motion is encouraged, which combines both vertical and lateral rotation control (i.e., rolling from prone to supine, then coming up into an upright position). When mastered, patients can always achieve a position in the water where they can breathe.

Phase 3: Control of Movement in Water

6. Use of upthrust. Patients are taught to control the amount of buoyant support the water provides. Examples include extending the arms and holding one's breath to encourage floating. Conversely, bringing the arms closer to the body and blowing air out promotes sinking.

7. Balance in stillness. Patients are taught to assume and hold a position in the water while turbulence challenges their steadiness.

8. Turbulent gliding. When able to assume and hold horizontal positions (i.e., supine), the therapist creates turbulence around the patient to move him or her through the water. This assisted movement readies the patient for more independent control of movement through the water.

Phase 4: Movement in Water

9. Basic progression. Before learning specific swimming strokes, patients are encouraged to move themselves through the water in the easiest manner possible. Usually bilateral, symmetric movements are attempted (i.e., elementary backstroke) before bilateral, asymmetric movements (i.e., back crawl stroke).

10. Swimming progression. Specific swimming strokes are approached. At this time, many therapists rely on principles from other schools of thought (e.g., American Red Cross Adapted Swimming Instruction) to promote skill.

Use for Patients with Neurologic Disorders

Using the Halliwick method for swimming instruction is ultimately therapeutic for all people because of the conditioning effects inherent in this form of exercise. It is particularly helpful for individuals with impairment and disability secondary to neurologic disorders. The approach can also be used to influence movement problems directly, for example, patients believed to be dominated by extensor movement patterns may benefit from gaining skill in vertical rotation control in an anterior direction (Figure 3-6). Such a movement helps the patient to actively control flexor musculature and inhibit extensor musculature. Skill gained through balance-in-stillness activities may carry over and influence postural stability during functional activities (Figure 3-7).

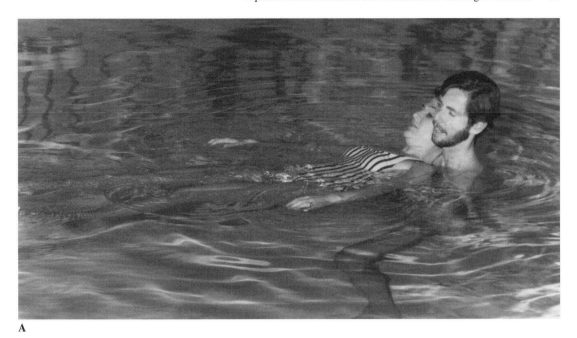

A

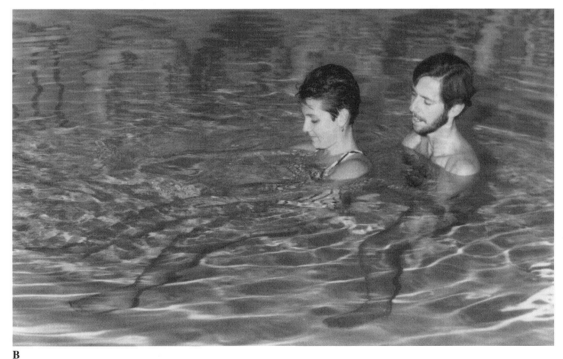

B

Figure 3-6. Using the Halliwick method, the therapist assists the patient to gain vertical rotation control in the water. Using her head to lead, the patient uses vertical rotation to move from a supine to a cube position.

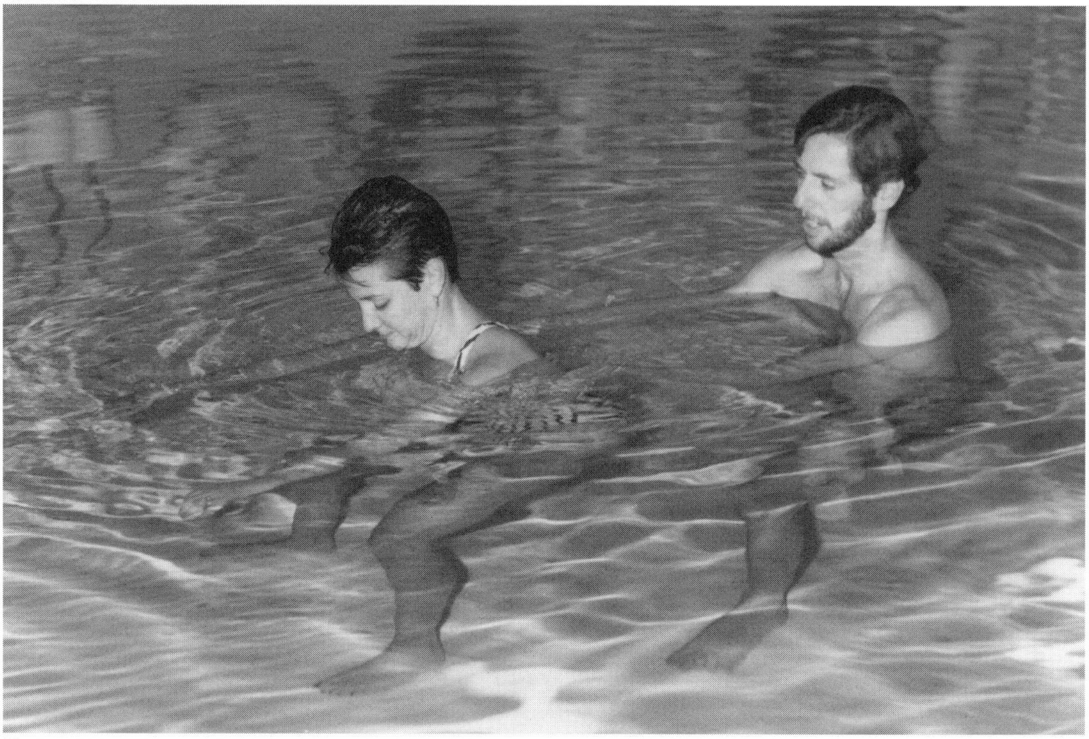

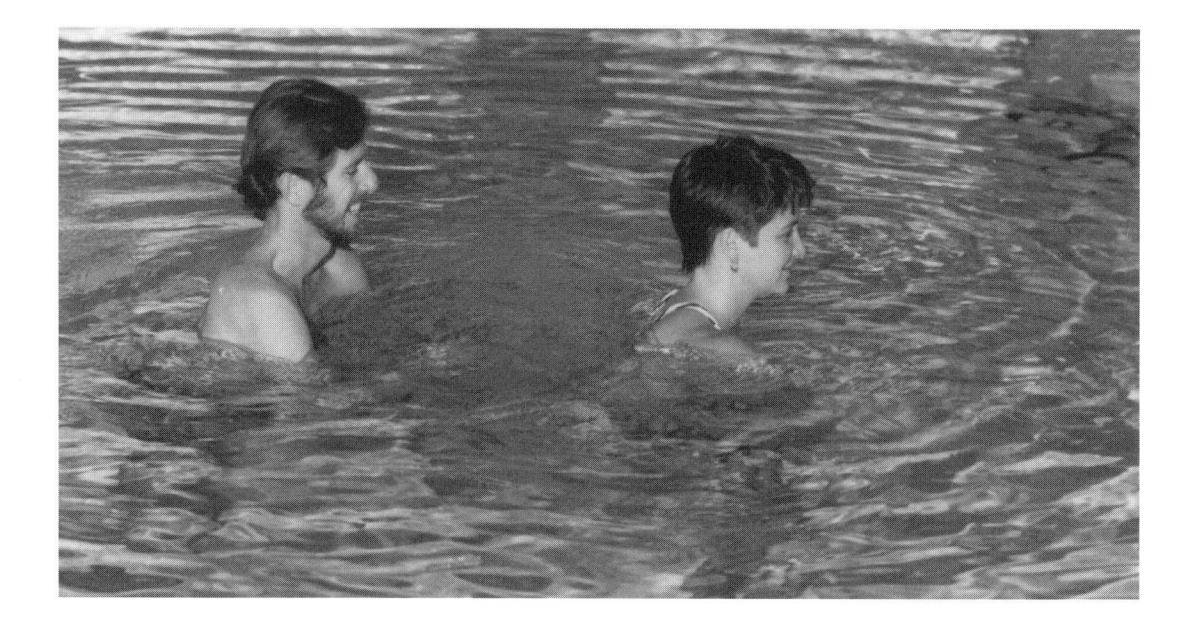

C

Figure 3-6. *(continued)*

Figure 3-7. Using the Halliwick method, the therapist follows a balance-in-stillness principle by creating turbulence behind the patient and challenging the patient's stability.

Table 3-2. General Principles of the Task-Type Training Approach

Work in the most shallow water tolerated.
Practice functional activities as a whole.
Systematically remove external stabilization provided for patients.
Encourage stabilizing contractions in upright positions with movement of selected body segments.
Encourage quick, reciprocal movement.
Encourage active movement problem solving.

Task-Type Training Approach

A task-type training approach (TTTA) for aquatic rehabilitation has been documented for patients who have survived a stroke [22]. For this book, the guidelines and principles of the TTTA are extended to the treatment of all patients with neurologic disorders. The TTTA can best be described as a task-oriented approach: Emphasis is placed on influencing the patient's disability by working in functional positions with functional activities. In addition, patients are encouraged to become active problem solvers of their movement difficulties as opposed to passive recipients of manual and verbal input from therapists. Notably, the TTTA is not a treatment technique but a set of principles to guide therapists in designing treatment programs for their patients' disabilities (Table 3-2). The general principles are as follows:

1. Work in the most shallow water tolerated. The buoyant support of the water allows patients to stand independently and move in a functional manner for the first time. Patients can actively and aggressively bring about positive influences on functional disabilities. The ultimate goal is for the functional improvement to carry over to gravity-influenced land activities; therefore, the effect of buoyant support should be systematically removed as patients demonstrate skill with functional activities. Performance indicators, such as the inability to maintain an erect trunk while standing or the inability to maintain knee extension in supporting lower extremities, may show that deeper water is better for functional activity practice.

2. Practice functional activities as a whole. Although some treatment programs address strengthening or stretching of specific body segments or facilitating specific movement patterns, the TTTA encourages practice of activities that are identical to or closely approximate the land functional activities to be improved. This principle is based on a specificity-of-training principle that a functional skill must be practiced to be learned [23,24]. When performed as a whole, the entire functional skill must be mastered, including control of moving body segments and appropriately graded contraction of stabilizing body segments.

3. Systematically remove external stabilization from patients. Holding onto the pool wall or the therapist's manual assistance may be necessary in the earlier stages of a TTTA. This externally applied stabilization should be quickly removed as patients gain independent control over the functional activity. Thus, the therapist minimizes the patient's dependence on outside support for functional skills.

4. Encourage stabilizing contractions in upright positions with movement of selected body segments. Vertical or upright positions (i.e., sitting, standing) are positions of function and should be used as much as possible. Stereotypical strategies for maintaining postural stability in upright positions have been identified [25]. Patients with neurologic disorders typically have difficulty using these strategies to maintain their balance, so they are encouraged to relearn these maneuvers in a safe but challenging environment, the water. As patients move their extremi-

ties in or above the water, their center of balance is challenged. Prevention of falling requires use of effective postural stability strategies (Figure 3-8). The patient is forced to solve problems actively to redevelop these strategies, with attention given to contracting the appropriate muscles, in the proper sequence, and with the appropriate force of contraction.

5. Encourage quick, reciprocal movement. After many types of neurologic insults, neural shock produces a period of inactivity in which many forms of deconditioning occur. Studies indicate that many patients with neurologic disorders have a predominance of slow-twitch muscle fibers in their skeletal muscles, indicating that a conversion from fast- to slow-twitch fibers has occurred [17,26]. Some believe that this muscle fiber change contributes to the slow, labored movement typically seen in patients with neurologic disorders [17,26]. Many functional activities require rhythmic, reciprocal movements along with quick movement changes to maximize the use of inertial forces. Movement in this manner ensures smooth and efficient execution of functional activities. Weakness, ROM limitations, and other voluntary movement deficits prevent patients with neurologic disorders from moving effectively in a gravity environment; the supportive and assistive properties of water dramatically increase the likelihood of their doing so. Therefore, whenever possible, quick, reciprocal movements should be practiced (e.g., marching in place, pedaling the legs while supine). Such practice may produce a conditioning effect that will positively influence the impairments that constrain patients with neurologic disorders to slow, labored movements.

6. Encourage active movement problem solving. Motor learning research suggests that healthy humans learn movement skills better when they actively participate in the learning process [23,27]. For example, when subjects are given less feedback on their performance and are required to practice many and varied activities, they must become more reliant on their own ability to critique and modify their performance, leading to more active participation. Studies of patients with neurologic disorders have come to similar conclusions. For this reason, patients should be encouraged to critique their performance and propose movement solutions to their problems. Open-ended questions, such as "How did you do that time?" and "How can you improve your next attempt?", should be used whenever possible. When working with patients with neurologic disorders in the pool, several factors may make the use of such principles difficult. Many patients with neurologic disorders have difficulty critiquing their performance because of physical (i.e., sensory) and cognitive (i.e., perceptual) impairments. In this case, the therapist must provide minimal guiding feedback regarding the patient's performance.

Some authors have discouraged the use of an aquatic environment for functional training of patients with neurologic disorders because of the distorted feedback to movement provided by the supportive and refractory properties of water [4,6]. Activities in water result in inaccurate visual and weight-bearing feedback. Although this is true, other properties of water (e.g., turbulence) heighten sensory feedback to movement, which may assist patients' motor problem solving [22].

CONCLUSION

Challenges to the delivery of care to patients with neurologic disorders encourage rehabilitation professionals to explore many approaches to neurorehabilitation. Anec-

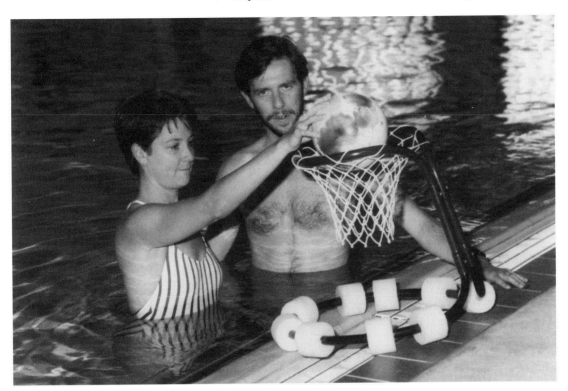

Figure 3-8. The patient practices using postural stability strategies while putting the ball into the basket.

dotally, aquatic rehabilitation has been effectively used to improve many impairment- and disability-oriented problems for these patients. Aquatic neurorehabilitation approaches must be carefully chosen and based on functional principles. Research is needed to examine the effectiveness of these approaches and study the carryover of aquatic therapeutic activities to land. Such endeavors will improve the delivery of aquatic rehabilitation to patients with neurologic disorders.

CASE STUDY

The patient is a 24-year-old male who sustained a traumatic brain injury in a motor vehicle accident 5 months ago. He is presently an outpatient at the rehabilitation center. He is alert and oriented, is able to follow simple directions, and he talks but is difficult to understand. He does appear to lack safety awareness. He has heterotopic bone in his right knee and both elbows. He has a thin build and is 6 ft, 4 in. tall.

Subjective Evaluation

The patient states that he has been living in his parents' one-story home since his accident. His family has a house on a nearby lake and he has always enjoyed swimming; he wants to walk again.

Objective Evaluation

Passive ROM	Right (degrees)	Left (degrees)
Shoulder flexion	90	105
Shoulder abduction	90	95
Elbow flexion	90	90
Elbow extension	–90	–35
Wrist flexion	WNL	WNL
Wrist extension	WNL	0
Hip flexion	70	80
Hip extension	–13	0
Hip abduction	10	15
Knee flexion	WNL	WNL
Knee extension	–30	0
Ankle dorsiflexion	–10	0

Active Movement

The patient exhibits active movement throughout his upper extremities through available ROM. He does move in a moderate flexor synergy pattern, however. He exhibits active movement throughout both lower extremities through available ROM with moderate influence of an extensor synergy pattern. He exhibits clonus in both ankles in standing.

Functional Activities

The patient performs standing pivot transfers with maximum to moderate assistance one time, requires minimal assistance with sitting balance, ambulates 25 ft with a platform walker, and needs maximum assistance three times to hold him upright and guide walker.

Gait Deviations

The patient can advance both lower extremities but requires assistance in stance on right lower extremity to extend knee. He also adducts both legs during swing.

Other

He exhibits poor sitting posture with forward head and flexed trunk. He requires constant verbal cues to sit erect and is unable to hold this position for more than 1 minute.

Impression

The patient is a good candidate for aquatic physical therapy because he is able to follow directions, is motivated, and is comfortable in the water. Treatment will be directed toward improving ROM and movement control at an impairment level and improving transfers, sitting, and gait at a disability level.

The patient's major problems are as follows:

1. Dependent for activities of daily living (ADL), including ambulation
2. Limited active and passive ROM
3. Voluntary movement deficits in all extremities
4. Poor sitting posture

Long-Term Goals (4 Weeks)

1. The patient is able to perform standing pivot transfer with minimal assistance one time. (In water, the patient will be able to perform an independent standing pivot transfer in 4-ft depth.)
2. The patient is able to ambulate 50 ft with rolling platform walker and moderate assistance one time. (In water, the patient is able to ambulate in 4-ft–deep water with moderate assistance one time with therapist standing at the patient's side, supporting the patient at the waist and holding onto the patient's right hand.)
3. The patient sits independently in 3-ft–deep water and can hold an erect posture with less than three verbal cues for 3 minutes.
4. Patient and family education is completed.

Plan

Patient will be seen three times a week for aquatic physical therapy, including therapeutic exercise, ADL training, and patient and family education. He will also be seen three times a week for physical therapy on land.

Treatment Program

General Considerations

Before beginning treatment with this patient, a thorough orientation to the program should be conducted for the patient and his family. The patient's lack of safety awareness is of great concern, and the therapist should prevent potential problems by setting firm ground rules to be followed while the patient is in the therapeutic pool setting. Because the patient's family does own a house on a lake, and they may be visiting on the weekends, basic water safety concepts should be discussed with the entire family. For example, the patient should be discouraged from participating in any water activity, whether recreational, exercise, or swimming, outside of the therapeutic setting until he has acquired basic swimming skills and has been approved for such activities by an appropriate professional. This discussion is important because families may try to duplicate activities they have observed at the therapeutic pool, unaware of the risks involved.

The patient's stature has both positive and negative implications for program planning. His height and thin build reduces the effects of buoyant support, which will make handling more difficult and provide less buoyancy-assisted movement for the patient. Conversely, the patient's increased body density may allow enough weight-bearing to inhibit hypertonicity and provide added sensory input during standing activities.

Treatment of Impairments and Disabilities

Water Shiatsu.   The use of WATSU with this patient can prove beneficial for several reasons. First, the stretching effects provided by the activities can positively influence the soft-tissue compliance of muscle and joint structures, resulting in increased active ROM and improved quality of voluntary muscle activity. Maneuvers particularly appropriate for this patient include the leg push (promoting hip extension), the thigh rock (promoting hip abduction), and the arm-leg rock (promoting hip flexion and stretches the anterior chest wall). Therapists should be aware, however, that these maneuvers may be hindered by and will have little effect on joint contractures resulting from heterotopic bone formation. The WATSU maneuvers used may need to be modified to accommodate these restrictions.

Another benefit provided by WATSU includes the tone reduction and relaxation provided by vestibular stimulation. When WATSU is applied in a slow, rhythmic manner, the steady movement stimulates vestibular receptors, which reduce general body muscle tone through the lateral vestibulospinal tract. Care should be taken to keep WATSU activities with this patient at slow, steady speeds. Quick, jerky movements may actually increase muscle tone.

WATSU is best applied early in the treatment session (i.e., the first 15 minutes). In this way, the increased ROM, relaxation, and reduced hypertonicity will contribute to success with the treatment activities to follow.

Bad Ragaz Ring Method.   Activities of the BRRM can be used with this patient to improve voluntary movement control. The therapist should select extremity exercise patterns that encourage movement away from the pathologic synergy patterns exhibited by the patient (i.e., flexor synergy in the upper extremities and extensor synergy in the lower extremities). Additionally, trunk exercise patterns can be used to improve dynamic and static trunk control. Specifically, the upper extremity pattern of shoulder flexion, abduction, and external rotation can be used to improve arm elevation without the influence of the flexor synergy pattern. Similarly, the lower extremity pattern of hip flexion, abduction, internal rotation, knee flexion, and ankle dorsiflexion can be used. This pattern also moves out of the predominant extensor synergy pattern and carries over to an improved swing phase of that leg during gait.

The trunk pattern of lateral trunk flexion with lower trunk and pelvic extension and rotation to one side (with bilateral hip extension) is beneficial for this patient. Improved control with these movements carries over to most antigravity functional skills (i.e., sitting, standing, ambulating).

Because voluntary movement deficits are present with this patient (i.e., synergistic movement patterns) emphasis should be placed on smooth controlled movement through the ROM. Less concern should be placed on generating resistance by moving quickly. A moderate number of sets with reduced repetitions (i.e., five sets of five repetitions of each exercise) may be best with this patient because fatigue usually reduces quality of movement. Such an exercise schedule allows frequent rest periods.

Halliwick Method.   Principles of the Halliwick method can be applied to the direct treatment of this patient's impairments and disabilities. Specifically, the disengagement principle can be applied to improving balance in standing. Early sessions include practice holding the cube position in water with the therapist's assistance through proximal handholds (i.e., support provided at the patient's trunk). Once the patient is able to hold this position without therapist support, he can be challenged by turbulence created around his body. As he becomes independent with this skill, the activity can be made more difficult by moving to a less stable position (i.e., the triangle). The position change may require reapplication of the therapist's support through handling. Ultimately, activities become more challenging until he assumes a stick position independently while turbulence is created around him.

Task-Type Training Approach.   Treatment to reduce disability can follow the principles of a TTTA and should be focused on three functional skills: sitting, transfers, and ambulation.

SITTING.   Sitting activities can begin in a water depth such that the patient is submerged no greater than midchest level. This is generally the shallowest area of the pool. External stabilization can be provided by the therapist's hand or a flotation device such as a large inner tube. As the patient gains skill in maintaining independent sitting balance, the external support should be gradually removed. For example, two small flotation rings can be used to progress from the large inner tube. The patient can then be asked to move the small rings in a variety of directions to challenge his ability to maintain sitting balance. These movements should be performed slowly at first and progress to quick reciprocal movements. Once the patient has progressed away from using any buoyant support, he can be challenged by engaging in a "pass-the-ball" game requiring use of the upper extremities. The game can be made progressively more difficult by introducing intertrial variability (i.e., passing the ball at different times, speeds, and locations at random).

TRANSFERS.   Two chairs can be placed in shallow water to practice standing pivot transfers. At first, the chairs can be placed beside and facing the pool wall. The patient uses the wall to stabilize as he executes the transfer. He can also use the therapist's outstretched arm for additional support. As the patient's skill improves, the activity can be practiced in progressively shallower water. External stabilization can be reduced by moving away from the wall. Intermediately, the patient can use a float (i.e., inner tube) for support during activity execution. Ultimately, the patient should perform the activity without any stabilizing support. Intertrial variability can be introduced by varying the height of the chairs or the distance between the two.

AMBULATION.   An early TTTA activity can include standing at the pool wall in chest-deep water. The patient holds onto the wall with both hands for support. Single-limb stance activities begin with the patient flexing one hip with the knee bent and returning to the pool floor. The therapist blocks the stance knee and provides support at the patient's stance hip if needed. When one leg up is achieved, the patient is asked to alternate lifts between legs to perform a marching activity. Encourage the patient to march as quickly as his skill allows. As soon as he demonstrates moderate skill with the activity, he should be asked to reposition so that his side is next to the pool wall. If he is able, ask him to kick the leg farthest from the wall with his knee extended. This activity not only strengthens the kicking leg but also challenges the patient's ability to stabilize throughout the stance leg and trunk.

As the patient progresses to taking steps, provide stabilization with the therapist's hand-held assistance or through some flotation device (i.e., kickboards, stabilizer bar, or inner tube). The hand-held assistance provided with the TTTA is different from that provided with more facilitation-oriented approaches, such as the

Halliwick method. With facilitation-oriented approaches, the therapist guides the patient to improve the quality of his movement. Hand-held assistance provided with the TTTA, however, is more fixed, supplying a stability point to be manipulated by the patient. Generally, the therapist's hand-held assistance is more stabilizing and should be applied first. Encourage the patient to increase his walking speed as his skill progresses. As he achieves independent ambulation, increase activity difficulty by moving to shallower water, adding upper extremity requirements (i.e., passing a ball) and introducing intertrial variability (i.e., changing directions and stopping and starting on command).

REFERENCES

1. Gordon J. Assumptions Underlying Physical Therapy Intervention: Theoretical and Historical Perspectives. In JH Carr, RB Shepherd, J Gordon, et al. (eds), Movement Science: Foundations for Physical Therapy in Rehabilitation. Rockville, MD: Aspen, 1987;1.
2. Horak FB. Assumptions Underlying Motor Control for Neurologic Rehabilitation. In J Lister (ed), Contemporary Management of Motor Control Problems: Proceedings of the II STEP Conference. Alexandria, VA: Foundation for Physical Therapy, 1990;11.
3. Skinner A, Thompson A (eds). Duffield's Exercise in Water (3rd ed). New York: Churchill Livingstone, 1983.
4. Davis BC, Harrison RA. Hydrotherapy in Practice. New York: Churchill Livingstone, 1988.
5. Campion MR. Hydrotherapy in Pediatrics. Oxford: Heinemann Medical Books, 1985.
6. Campion MR. Adult Hydrotherapy: A Practical Approach. Oxford: Heinemann Medical Books, 1990.
7. Gehlsen GM, Grigsby SA, Winant DM. Effects of an aquatic fitness program on the muscular strength and endurance of patients with multiple sclerosis. Phys Ther 1984;64:653.
8. Garvey LA. Spinal cord injury and aquatics. Clin Manage 1991;11:21.
9. Hurley R, Lyons-Olski E, Sweetman NA, et al. Neurology and aquatic therapy. Clin Manage 1991;11:26.
10. Taylor EW, Morris DM, Shaddeau S, et al. The effects of water walking on hemiplegic gait. Aquatic Phys Ther Rep 1992;1:10.
11. Schumacher K. Classification of stroke problems and the use of standard terminology in the care of persons with stroke. Neurol Rep 1991;15:4.
12. Taub E. Motor behavior following deafferentation in the developing and motorically mature monkey. Adv Behav Biol 1976;18:675.
13. Evarts EV, Shinoda Y, Wise SP. Neurophysiological Approaches to Higher Brain Function. New York: Wiley, 1984.
14. Shik M, Orlovsky GM. Neurophysiology of locomotor automatism. Physiol Rev 1976;56:465.
15. Dull H. WATSU: Freeing the Body in Water. Harbin Hot Springs, CA: Harbin Springs Publishing, 1993.
16. Craik RL. Abnormalities of Motor Behavior. In MJ Lister (ed), Contemporary Management of Motor Control Problems: Proceedings of the II STEP Conference. Alexandria, VA: Foundation for Physical Therapy, 1990;155.
17. Ballantine B. Factors contributing to voluntary movement deficits and spasticity following cerebral vascular accidents. Neurol Rep 1991;15:15.
18. Boyle AM. The Bad Ragaz ring method. Physiotherapy 1981;67:265.
19. Sahrmann S, Norton BJ. The relationship of voluntary movement to spasticity in the upper motor neuron syndrome. Ann Neurol 1977;2:460.
20. Martin J. The Halliwick method. Physiotherapy 1981;67:288.
21. Campion MR. Water Activity Based on the Halliwick Method. In A Skinner, A Thompson (eds), Duffield's Exercise in Water (3rd ed). London: Bailliere Tindall, 1983;180.
22. Morris DM. Aquatic rehabilitation for the treatment of neurologic disorders. J Back Musculoskel Rehabil 1994;4:297.

23. Winstein CJ. Designing Practice for Motor Learning: Clinical Implications. In MJ Lister (ed), Contemporary Management of Motor Control Problems: Proceedings of the II STEP Conference. Alexandria, VA: Foundation for Physical Therapy, 1990;65.

24. Winstein CJ, Gardner ER, McNeal DR, et al. Standing balance training: effect on balance and locomotion in hemiparetic adults. Arch Phys Med Rehabil 1989;70:755.

25. Horak FB, Schumway-Cook A. Clinical Implications of Postural Control Research. In PW Duncan (ed), Balance. Alexandria, VA: American Physical Therapy Association, 1990;105.

26. McComas AJ, Sica RE, Upton AR, et al. Functional changes in motoneurons of hemiparetic patients. J Neurol Neurosurg Psychiatry 1973;36:183.

27. Schmidt RA. Motor Learning Principles for Physical Therapy. In MJ Lister (ed), Contemporary Management of Motor Control Problems: Proceedings of the II STEP Conference. Alexandria, VA: Foundation for Physical Therapy, 1990;49.

4

Spine Pain: Aquatic Rehabilitation Strategies

Andrew J. Cole, Marilou Moschetti,
Richard A. Eagleston, and Steven A. Stratton

Physicians tell many spine patients to swim for rehabilitation, exercise, and pain management, but the role that the aquatic environment plays in spine rehabilitation has not been explored fully. Water's unique properties make it ideal for rehabilitating patients with spinal pain, and various methods may be used to integrate water-based programs into comprehensive training regimens.

BACKGROUND

In the United States, aquatic activity is the most common participation sport and is an extremely popular exercise for recreation, competition, and rehabilitation [1]. More than 26,000 people are involved with U.S. Masters Swimming, and more than 2,000 centers use aquatic techniques for rehabilitative purposes (U.S. Masters Swimming, personal communication, 1993). The rising popularity of aquatic activities has resulted in increasing numbers of spinal and associated musculoskeletal injuries. Land exercises, swimming, and inappropriate aquatic rehabilitation programs can cause new spinal injuries or exacerbate pre-existing spinal disorders, but properly designed aquatic programs can help rehabilitate patients with spinal injuries. Aquatic stabilization techniques and swimming programs can be used with aggressive, comprehensive, land-based spine-stabilization programs or as the sole rehabilitative tools [2]. The success or failure of aquatic therapy candidates is not determined by swimming skills alone because swim-stroke proficiency is not a model for successful treatment.

DIAGNOSIS AND TREATMENT

The workup and diagnosis of spinal pain require a thorough understanding of anatomy, physiology, and activity-specific functional biomechanics. After carefully obtaining a history, with close attention to the specific mechanism of injury, a physi-

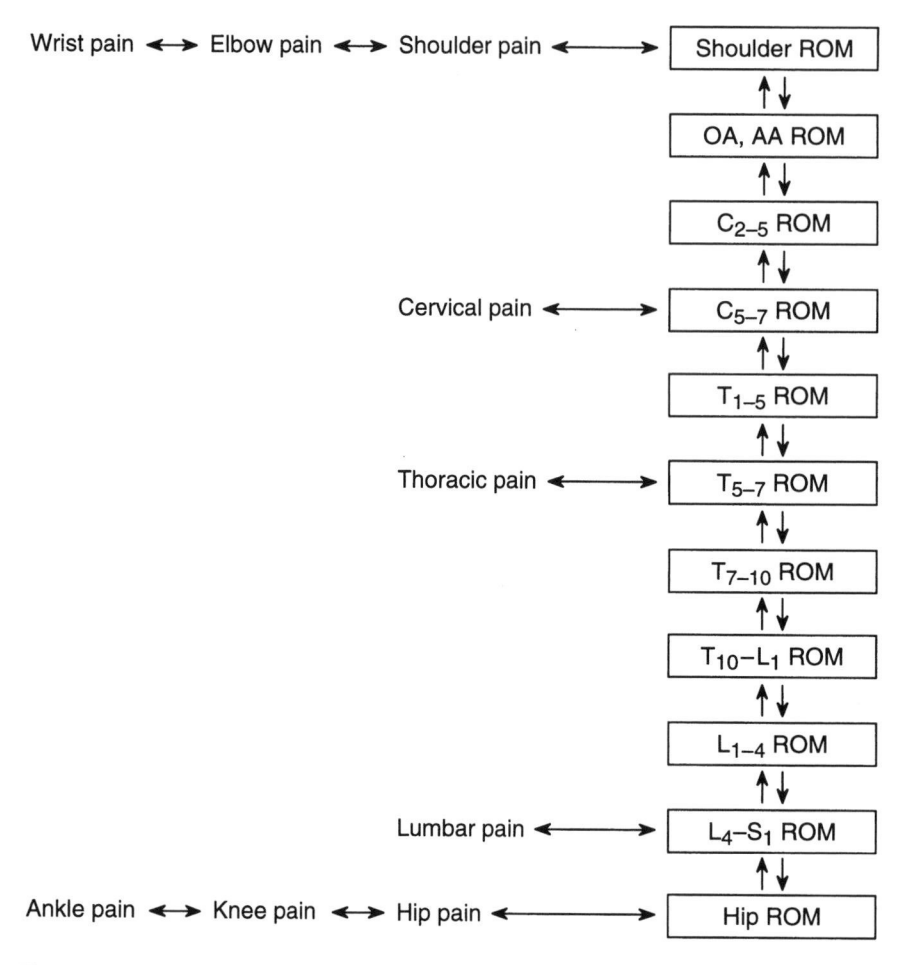

Figure 4-1. Peripheral joint dysfunction can set off a motion cascade throughout the spinal axis; conversely, spine dysfunction can create peripheral joint dysfunction. (ROM = range of motion; C = cervical; T = thoracic; AA = atlantoaxial; L = lumbar; S = sacral; OA = occipitoatlantal.) (Courtesy of AquaTechnics Consulting Group, Inc., Aptos, CA.)

cian performs a thorough yet directed neurologic and musculoskeletal examination of the injured structure and its contiguous supporting elements. A functional evaluation is conducted in which the patient reproduces a painful motion. Finally, ancillary testing is ordered and the correct final diagnosis is confirmed.

An understanding of anatomy and stroke-specific functional biomechanics allows thorough treatment plans and complete rehabilitation programs to be developed. A rehabilitation program addresses the primary injury, whether spinal or peripheral joint, as well as secondary sites of dysfunction [3–6].

Recognition of the functional relationship between the spine and peripheral joints is critical to ensure optimal treatment outcomes. Peripheral joint dysfunction can set off a cascading series of motion changes throughout the spinal axis. The cervicothoracic and thoracolumbar transition zones, in particular, are commonly affected because they are the junctions of the more mobile and less mobile sections of the spine [7]. Figure 4-1 presents the motion cascade originally described by Cole and Herring [8]. In a swimmer, for example, a shoulder injury, such as rotator cuff ten-

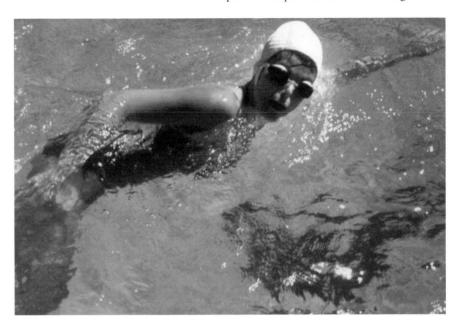

Figure 4-2. Crane breathing during the freestyle stroke is a biomechanical adaptation that improves access to air by increasing capital and cervical spine extension and rotation. Such breathing can occur for a variety of reasons, the most common being poor body roll. (Courtesy of AquaTechnics Consulting Group, Inc., Aptos, CA.)

dinitis, results in guarding and decreased range of shoulder motion [3,8–11]. The swimmer's arm cannot abduct and extend as it would [12] during normal recovery, resulting in decreased body roll, increased lumbar segmental motion, and an abnormally low head position from which to breathe [2]. Compensatory adaptive changes then occur. Such changes include crane breathing (increased cervical suboccipital extension and rotation, cervical extension [C2–C7], and cervical rotation [C2–C7]) (Figure 4-2), as well as more extension and rotation from C3 to C5 [2]. To compensate, the C5–T1 segment becomes hypomobile, and mid- and low-cervical pain results. Compensatory hypermobility begins from T2 to T5 and hypomobility from T5 to T7 and T10 to L1. Primary cervical, thoracic, and lumbar injuries and pain influence the spinal axis in a similar fashion. Hip [13], pelvis, and lumbar spine pain result in hypomobility at L4–S1 and ultimately at the T10–L1 transition zone. Adaptive changes proceed up the axis and may set the stage for compensatory changes in shoulder mechanics that eventually cause a shoulder injury. Identifying the initial injury is important so that treatment can eliminate that problem as well as secondary compensatory sites of dysfunction [3,8,14].

When prescribing rehabilitation plans, it is important to recognize that physiologic and psychological needs vary among patient populations. Highly competitive athletes, for example, require alternative training regimens during their rehabilitation programs to maintain peak flexibility, strength, and aerobic conditioning. Recreational athletes may be more flexible in this regard. Competitive athletes require specific training schedules and goals to compete effectively during particular athletic seasons, but the needs of weekend athletes are usually not as rigorous. Specific patient goals are met by tailoring workups and rehabilitation programs to athletic

Table 4-1. Benefits of Aquatic Stabilization Programs

Minimization of segmental trunk motion and shear forces
Reinforcement of lumbar control
Encouragement of hip, knee, and ankle propulsion
Development of head and neck stability
Establishment of arm control and strength

demand levels. Finally, changes in training routines and sports-specific mechanics require close cooperation of physicians, patients, therapists, and coaches [15].

REHABILITATION PROGRAMS

The aquatic rehabilitation programs reviewed here are based on dynamic lumbar, thoracic, and cervical stabilization techniques that have been described for land programs [16,17]. Dynamic land-based stabilization training is a specific type of therapeutic exercise that can help patients gain dynamic control of segmental spine forces; eliminate repetitive injury to motion segments, that is, discs, zygapophyseal joints, and related structures; encourage healing of injured motion segments; and possibly alter the degenerative process. The underlying premise is that motion segments and supporting soft tissues react to minimize applied stresses and reduce risk of injury [16,17]. The goals of aquatic stabilization exercise and swimming programs incorporate these elements but take into account the unique properties of water so that the risk of spinal injury is reduced. Aquatic stabilization programs help to develop patients' flexibility, strength, and body mechanics so that a smooth transition to aquatic stabilization swimming programs or other spine-stabilized aquatic activities may occur. Such programs can help first-time swimmers and patients who previously swam (Table 4-1) [2,8,11,18,19].

REHABILITATION ENVIRONMENT: LAND VS. WATER

Accurate diagnosis of patients' spinal injuries and observation of their initial responses to land-based or aquatic stabilization programs help to determine further treatment with therapeutic exercises. A transition from dry to wet exercise conditions eliminates dry-land risks, establishes a supportive training environment, provides a new therapeutic activity, decreases the risk of peripheral joint injury, and allows a return to prior activity. Moving from dry to wet environments also should be considered if patients cannot tolerate axial or gravitational loads, if they require increased support in the presence of a strength or proprioceptive deficit [20], or if they are at risk of a compression fracture due to decreased bone density [21]. Remaining in a water-supported environment is appropriate if a dry environment exacerbates symptoms or if patients prefer water. Transition from a wet to a dry environment should occur if patients are doing well in the water but must return to land to meet functional training needs efficiently and attain their ultimate competitive goals [18,22]. Table 4-2 lists specific contraindications for aquatic rehabilitation [11,23,24].

Table 4-2. Contraindications for Aquatic Rehabilitation

Fever
Cardiac failure
Urinary infections
Bowel or bladder incontinence
Open wounds
Infectious diseases
Contagious skin conditions
Excessive fear of water
Uncontrolled seizures
Colostomy bag or catheter used by patient
Cognitive or functional impairment that creates a hazard to the patient or others in pool
Severely weakened or deconditioned state that poses a safety hazard
Extremely poor endurance
Severely decreased range of motion that limits function and poses a safety hazard

Source: AquaTechnics Consulting Group, Inc., Aptos, CA.

Spinal rehabilitation programs offer advantages that are directly related to the intrinsic properties of water—namely, buoyancy, resistance, viscosity, hydrostatic pressure, temperature, turbulence, and refraction. We have described these properties elsewhere [2,11,18,25,26]. Graded elimination of gravitational forces through buoyancy allows patients to train with decreased yet variable axial loads and shear forces. In essence, water increases the safety margin of patient postural error by decreasing the compressive and shear forces on the spine. Motion velocity can be controlled by water resistance, viscosity, buoyancy, and training devices. Buoyancy increases the range of training positions. The psychological outlook of swimmers may be enhanced because rehabilitation occurs in their competitive environment. Many believe water reduces pain because of the sensory overload generated by hydrostatic pressure, temperature, and turbulence [19,27–40].

AQUATIC SPINE-STABILIZATION TECHNIQUES

The spine-stabilization principles discussed for land programs also apply to aquatic programs. Certain exercises that can be performed on land cannot be reproduced in water and vice versa. Aquatic programs can be designed for patients who cannot train on land and for those whose land training has reached a plateau. Richard Eagleston first described aquatic stabilization in 1989 [41].

We have developed eight core aquatic stabilization exercises with four levels of difficulty that provide graded training of stabilization skills [2,11,18,25,26]. Programs must be customized to meet the needs of each patient's unique spinal pathology, related musculoskeletal dysfunctions, and comfort with the aquatic environment. Also, patients who have had joint replacements require particular care during positioning in the water, because the replacements can change the center of buoyancy and may cause patients to sink due to high specific gravity [42]. When one program is mastered, a more advanced program is provided. Eventually, if a patient wants to begin a swimming program, a series of transitional aquatic stabilization exercises are initiated. These help to establish a spine-stabilized swimming style that minimizes the risk of further spinal injury and helps to maximize swimming performance [18,25].

Wall Sit

The wall sit exercise develops isometric strength primarily in the quadriceps and hamstring groups. It also trains abdominal muscles to hold the appropriate neutral spine posture [11,18,25].

- Level I: Supported by the pool wall, the patient maintains the vertical position with hips and knees in 90-degree flexion. This position is held for 1 minute (Figure 4-3).
- Level II: The patient holds the level 1 position for 2 minutes.
- Level III: The patient holds the position for 3 minutes.
- Level IV: The patient holds the position for 5 minutes.

Modified Superman

The modified Superman trains ipsilateral hip flexors, extensors, and contralateral gluteus medius and increases isometric strength in abdominal and paraspinal stabilizers [11,18,25].

- Level I: Facing the pool wall, the patient stands and holds on to the edge of the pool with both hands. Movement is unilateral, one leg at a time, with the knee flexed at 45 degrees. The hip is actively extended to 20 degrees and then returned to the neutral position. The movement pattern continues for 60 seconds at 50% of maximum velocity (Figure 4-4).
- Level II: Level II is performed exactly like level I, but the knee is maintained in full extension and the movement pattern continues for 2 minutes at 70% of maximum velocity (Figure 4-5).
- Level III: Level III is performed exactly like level II, but a 3-lb cuff is applied to each ankle. This movement pattern continues for 2 minutes at 50% of maximum velocity (Figure 4-6).
- Level IV: Level IV is performed exactly like level III, but the pattern continues for 3–5 minutes at 85% of maximum velocity.

Water Walking Forward

Water walking forward isometrically strengthens the abdominal muscles and muscle groups that maintain proper posture. Isotonic strengthening occurs in muscles that are dynamically involved in gait [11,18,25].

- Level I: The patient begins in the standing position, unsupported, with the water depth at the xiphoid level. Elbows are extended with the palms at the sides and forward. The patient water walks for 3 minutes at 50% of maximum velocity (Figure 4-7).
- Level II: Level II provides an incrementally greater challenge for all muscle groups described in level I. The arms are abducted to 45 degrees and hand

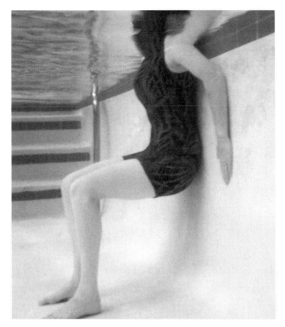

Figure 4-3. The wall sit develops isometric strength, primarily in the quadriceps and hamstring groups. Abdominal muscles are trained to hold the appropriate neutral spine posture. (Courtesy of AquaTechnics Consulting Group, Inc., Aptos, CA.)

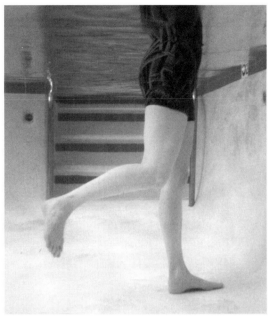

Figure 4-4. Modified Superman level I. (Courtesy of AquaTechnics Consulting Group, Inc., Aptos, CA.)

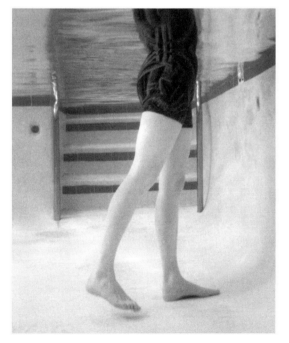

Figure 4-5. Modified Superman level II. (Courtesy of AquaTechnics Consulting Group, Inc., Aptos, CA.)

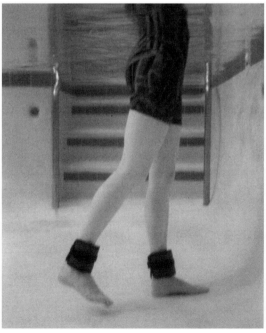

Figure 4-6. Modified Superman levels III and IV. (Courtesy of AquaTechnics Consulting Group, Inc., Aptos, CA.)

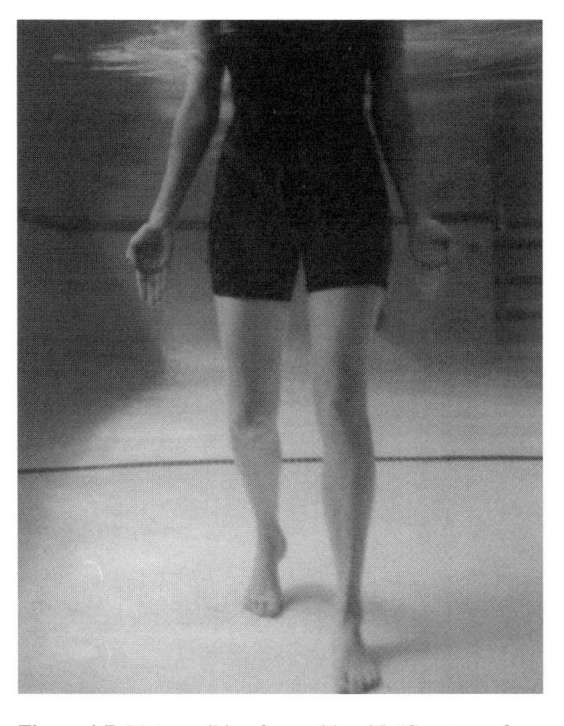

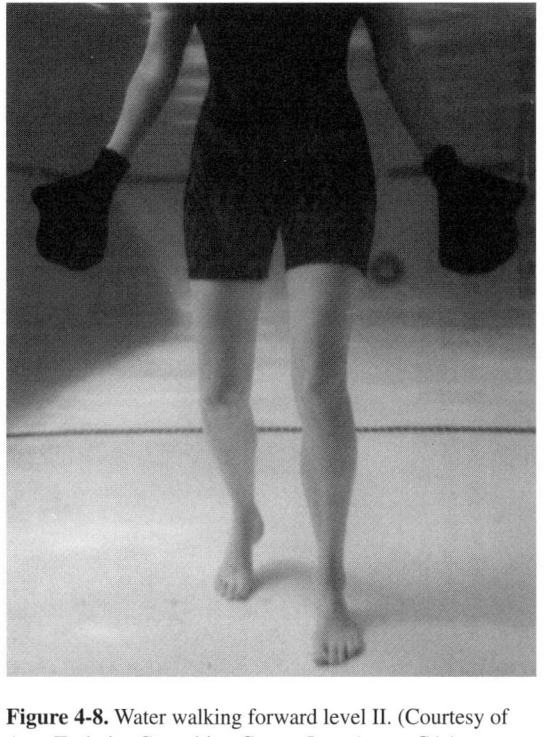

Figure 4-7. Water walking forward level I. (Courtesy of AquaTechnics Consulting Group, Inc., Aptos, CA.)

Figure 4-8. Water walking forward level II. (Courtesy of AquaTechnics Consulting Group, Inc., Aptos, CA.)

mitts are used. The patient walks for 5 minutes at 70% of maximum velocity (Figure 4-8).

- Level III: Level III further enhances resistive training. Hand paddles are used, and the patient walks for 10 minutes at 85% of maximum velocity (Figure 4-9).
- Level IV: The patient walks forward and backward with water shoes or 3-lb ankle weights, or both. A piece of Plexiglas (36 × 24 in.) or a kickboard held vertically beneath the water surface increases the resistance. The exercise is performed for 10 minutes at a velocity of 90–100% of maximum velocity (Figure 4-10).

Water Walking Backward

Water walking backward, like the previous exercise, provides similar strengthening, but with greater emphasis on isometric paraspinal muscle conditioning [11,18,25].

- Level I: The patient begins in the standing position, unsupported, with the water depth at the xiphoid level. Elbows are kept extended with the palms at the sides and forward. The patient water walks backward for 3 minutes at 50% of maximum velocity (Figure 4-11).
- Level II: Level II provides an incrementally greater challenge for all muscle groups described in level I. The arms are abducted to 45 degrees and hand mitts

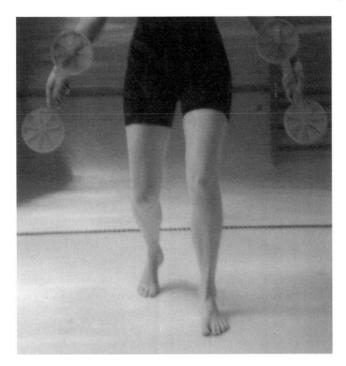

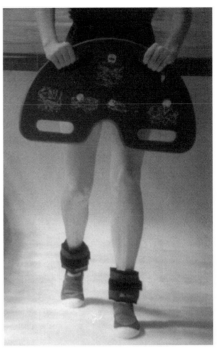

Figure 4-9. Water walking forward level III. (Courtesy of AquaTechnics Consulting Group, Inc., Aptos, CA.)

Figure 4-10. Water walking forward level IV. (Courtesy of AquaTechnics Consulting Group, Inc., Aptos, CA.)

are used. The patient walks backward for 5 minutes at 70% of maximum velocity (Figure 4-12).

- Level III: Level III further enhances resistive training. Hand paddles are used, and the patient walks backward for 10 minutes at 85% of maximum velocity (Figure 4-13).
- Level IV: The patient walks forward and backward with water shoes or 3-lb ankle weights, or both. A piece of Plexiglas (36 × 24 in.) or a kickboard held vertically beneath the water surface increases the resistance. The exercise is performed for 10 minutes at a velocity of 90–100% of maximum velocity (Figure 4-14).

Supine Sculling

Supine sculling simultaneously initiates strengthening in the upper- and lower-extremity muscle groups. Posterior and anterior muscle groups of the lower extremities, gluteals, shoulder complex, and paraspinals are incrementally challenged [11,18,25].

- Level I: The patient wears a flotation jacket to support the torso and a flotation collar for the neck while being maintained in a supine, supported position by the therapist. The upper extremities simultaneously perform a sculling figure-eight movement at the hip, while the lower extremities initiate a flutter kick.

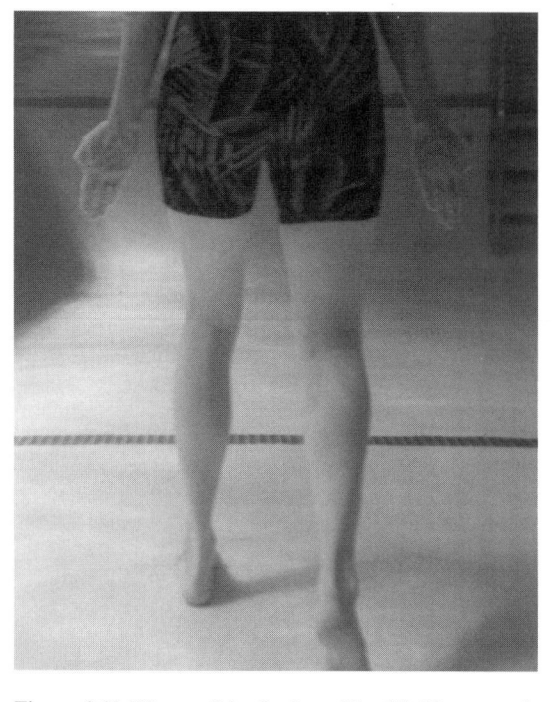

Figure 4-11. Water walking backward level I. (Courtesy of AquaTechnics Consulting Group, Inc., Aptos, CA.)

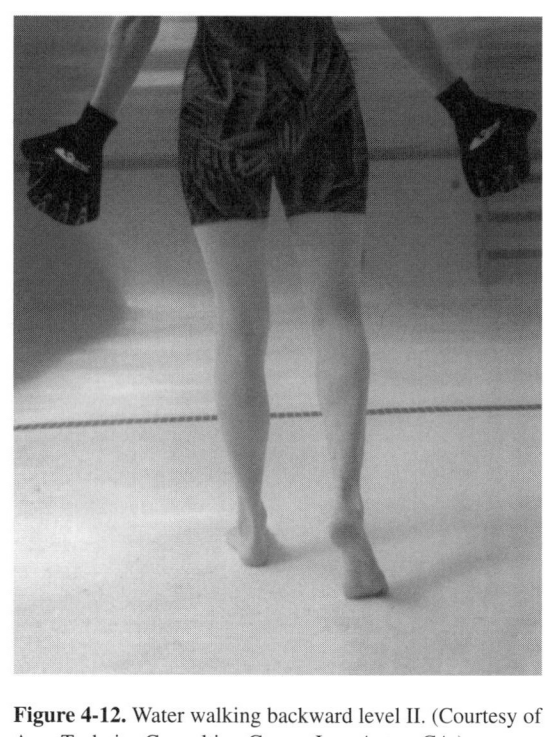

Figure 4-12. Water walking backward level II. (Courtesy of AquaTechnics Consulting Group, Inc., Aptos, CA.)

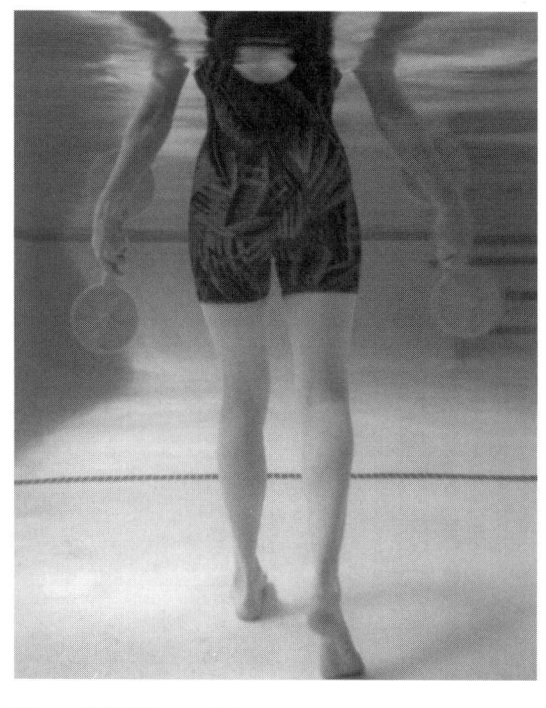

Figure 4-13. Water walking backward level III. (Courtesy of AquaTechnics Consulting Group, Inc., Aptos, CA.)

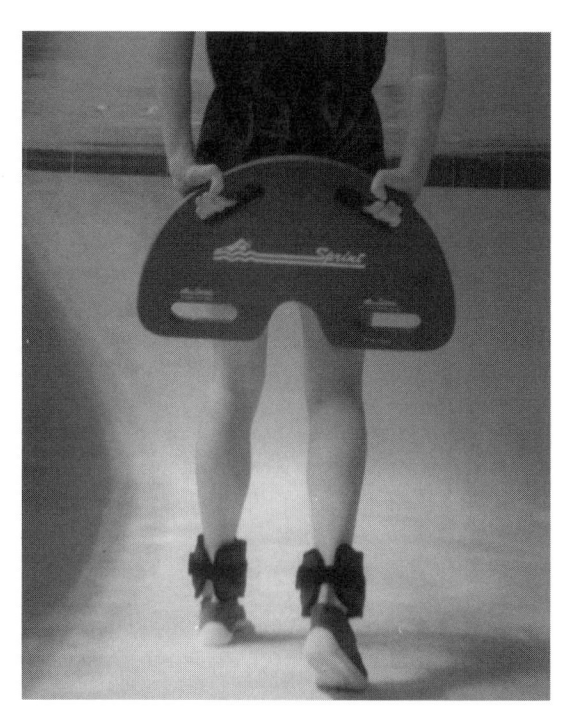

Figure 4-14. Water walking backward level IV. (Courtesy of AquaTechnics Consulting Group, Inc., Aptos, CA.)

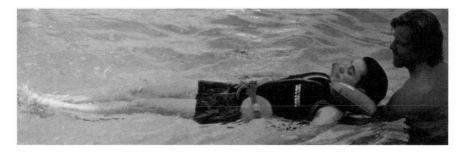

Figure 4-15. Supine sculling level I. (Courtesy of AquaTechnics Consulting Group, Inc., Aptos, CA.)

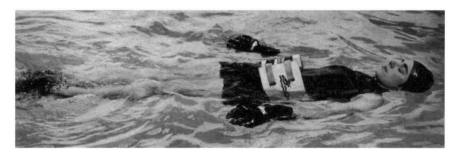

Figure 4-16. Supine sculling level II. (Courtesy of AquaTechnics Consulting Group, Inc., Aptos, CA.)

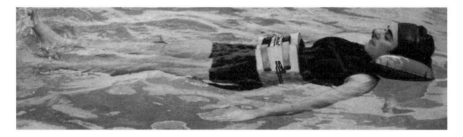

Figure 4-17. Supine sculling level III. (Courtesy of AquaTechnics Consulting Group, Inc., Aptos, CA.)

This exercise is performed for 1 minute at 50% of maximum velocity (Figure 4-15).
- Level II: A flotation belt is substituted for the flotation jacket, and the cervical flotation support is maintained. The therapist supervises but does not support the patient. Arms are abducted to 40 degrees, and the flutter is increased in intensity. This exercise is performed for 3 minutes at 70% of maximum velocity (Figure 4-16).
- Level III: Hand mitts and short fins are added. The flotation belt continues to be used, but the cervical support device is eliminated. This exercise pattern is performed for 5 minutes at 85% of maximum velocity (Figure 4-17).

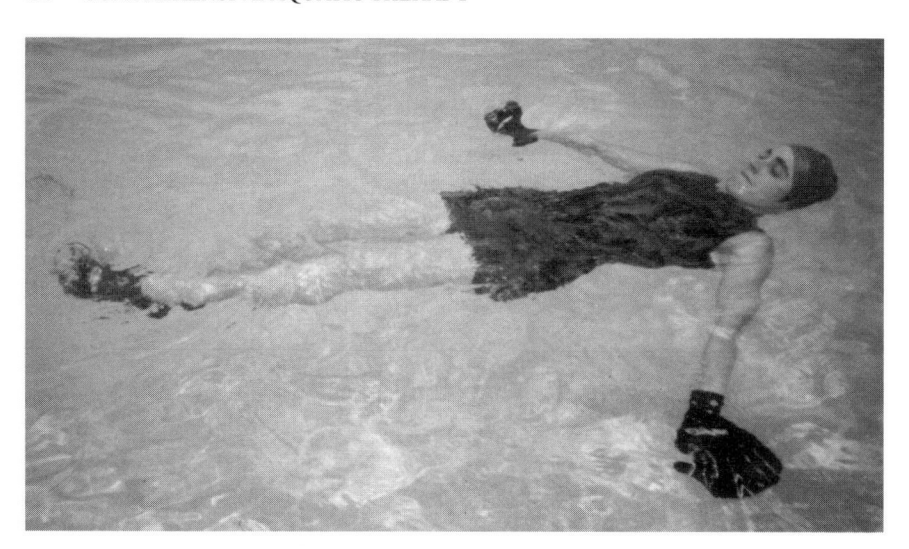

Figure 4-18. Supine sculling level IV. (Courtesy of AquaTechnics Consulting Group, Inc., Aptos, CA.)

- Level IV: The flotation device is eliminated. Short-blade fins and hand mitts are used. Sculling and kicking are performed for 30 seconds followed by 15 seconds of rest. The exercise is performed at 90–100% of maximum velocity; 12 sets are performed (Figure 4-18).

Wall Crunch

Wall crunch exercises train muscles activated in the wall sit and additionally challenge contralateral gluteals, ipsilateral hip flexors, rotational abdominals, and paraspinals [11,18,25].

- Level I: The patient stands with the spine against the pool wall and flexes one hip to 90 degrees with the knee at 90-degree flexion. One hand provides isometric resistance, and the isometric contraction is held for 5 seconds. Ten repetitions at 50% of maximum velocity are performed (Figure 4-19).
- Level II: The patient stands with the spine against the pool wall and the arms hooked over the pool ledge and simultaneously flexes both hips to 90 degrees with knees at 90-degree flexion. The position is held for 10 seconds; 10 repetitions at 70% of maximum velocity are performed (Figure 4-20).
- Level III: The patient stands in the same position as level II and flexes both hips simultaneously to 90 degrees with the knees at full extension. Three-pound weights are attached to the ankles. The position is held for 10 seconds. Twenty repetitions at 50% of maximum velocity are performed (Figure 4-21).
- Level IV: This level is performed the same as level III; however, there is no isometric hold. The motion is continuous for 3 minutes at 50% of maximum velocity.

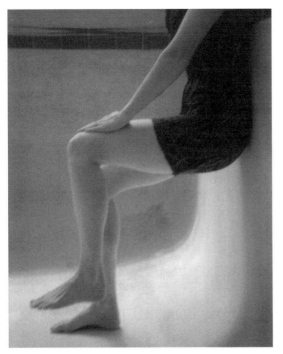

Figure 4-19. Wall crunch level I. (Courtesy of AquaTechnics Consulting Group, Inc., Aptos, CA.)

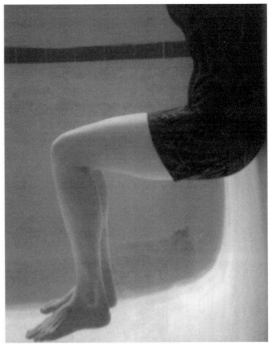

Figure 4-20. Wall crunch level II. (Courtesy of AquaTechnics Consulting Group, Inc., Aptos, CA.)

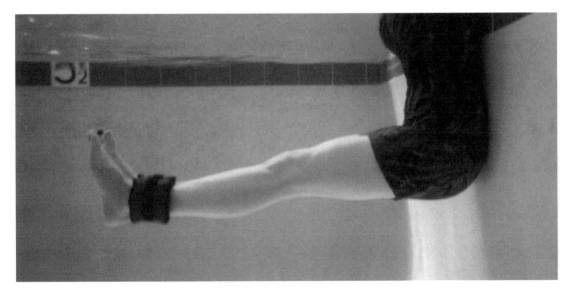

Figure 4-21. Wall crunch levels III and IV. (Courtesy of AquaTechnics Consulting Group, Inc., Aptos, CA.)

Quadruped

Quadruped is performed in the prone position, with the patient using a snorkel and mask to avoid the struggle for air while training arm and leg mechanics. A patient who is unfamiliar with the proper use of a snorkel and mask may be taught by a therapist in shallow water. The patient must perform all skills comfortably before proceeding. The patient must perform correct recovery from a prone position to a standing position. The therapist should not leave the patient unattended while using this equipment in the therapy pool [11,18,25].

Quadruped level I activities (legs only) challenge lumbar spine stabilizer groups isometrically and lower extremity hip flexors and extensors isotonically.

Level I quadruped activities (arms only) challenge lumbar spine stabilizer groups isometrically and upper extremity shoulder groups that reproduce flexion and extension isotonically.

- Level I: The patient begins in a semisupported prone position with a flotation belt at hip level. The therapist supports the legs and hips. The patient moves the arms simultaneously, with the elbows extended, from 0-degree to 180-degree forward flexion. This motion is performed for 1 minute at 50% of maximum velocity (Figure 4-22A). Next, the therapist supports the arms and instructs the patient simultaneously to move the legs from 0-degree hip position to 90-degree hip- and knee-flexed position (Figure 4-22B). This motion is performed for 1 minute at 50% of maximum velocity.
- Level II: The flotation device is removed, and the therapist supports the patient's hips. Alternating arm movements are performed in a pattern similar to level I for 3 minutes at 50% of maximum velocity (Figure 4-23A). The legs are then trained in an alternating pattern through the same range of motion as in level I (Figure 4-23B). This occurs for 3 minutes at 50% of maximum velocity.
- Level III: Level III increases the training intensity by requiring greater independence during activity. Therapist support is removed, but a flotation vest is used (Figure 4-24). The patient performs simultaneous, alternating upper- and lower-extremity patterns, as in level II, for 3 minutes at 70% of maximum velocity.
- Level IV: Weights are added to ankles and wrists for an additional challenge, and a flotation device is placed at the waist to prevent sinking (Figure 4-25). The movement pattern is the same as that of level III, but it continues for 5 minutes at 70% of maximum velocity.

When the patient can perform the quadruped, the log roll swim (a transition exercise to spine-stabilized swimming) is introduced.

Log-Roll Swim

Log-roll swim teaches spine-stabilized movement, thus eliminating segmental rotation through the spinal axis. The patient, supported at the hip with a small flotation belt, uses a snorkel and mask to ease breathing. The therapist may fix strapping tape to the lumbar spine to give proprioceptive cues and to help to avoid segmental spine movement [11,18,25].

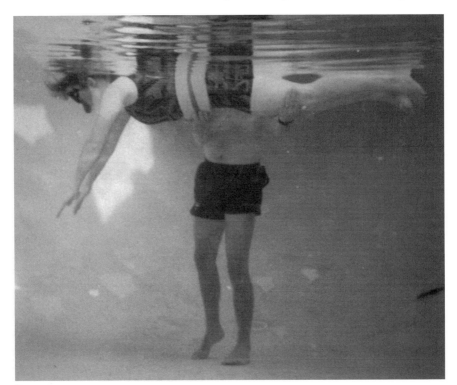

A

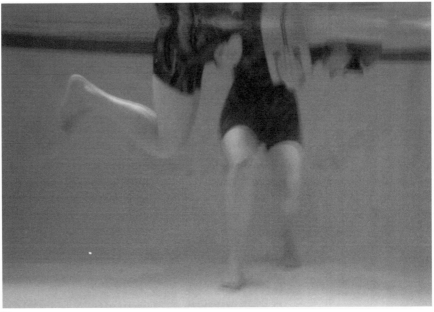

B

Figure 4-22. Quadruped level I. (Courtesy of AquaTechnics Consulting Group, Inc., Aptos, CA.)

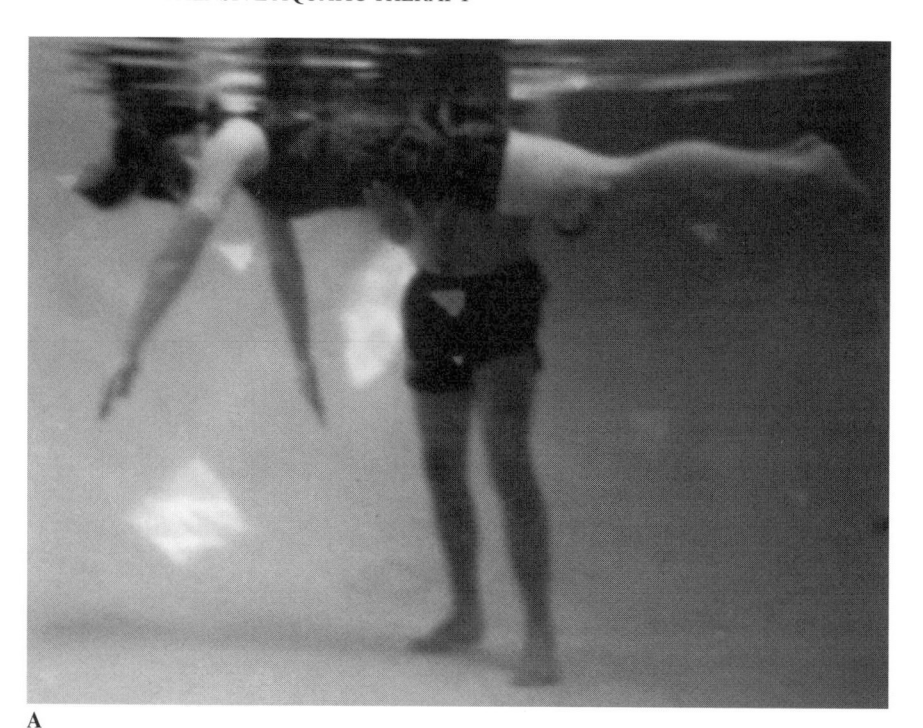

A

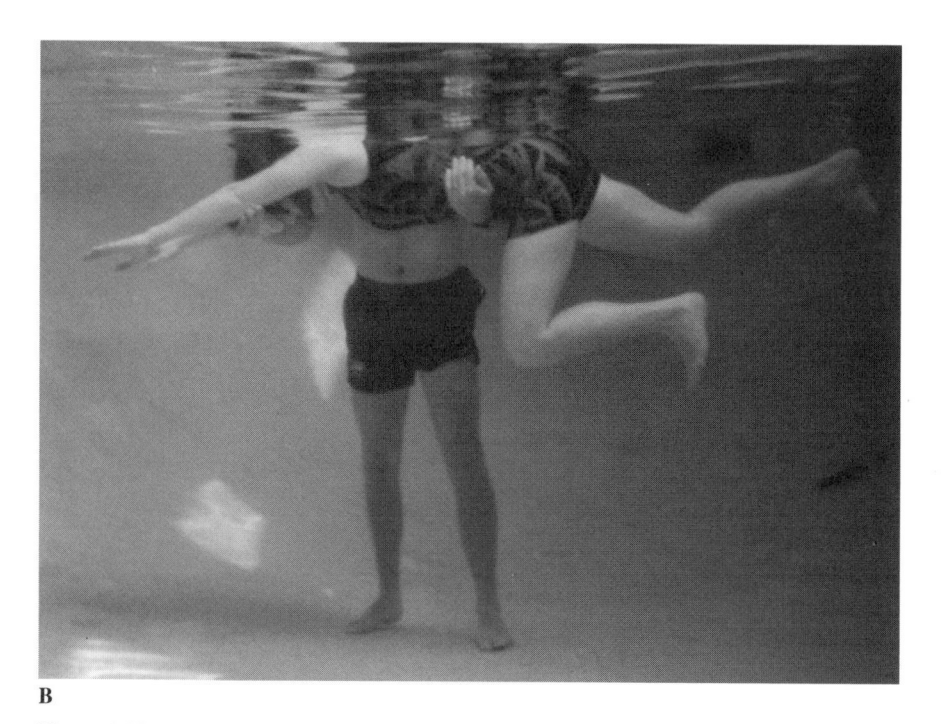

B

Figure 4-23. Quadruped level II. (Courtesy of AquaTechnics Consulting Group, Inc., Aptos, CA.)

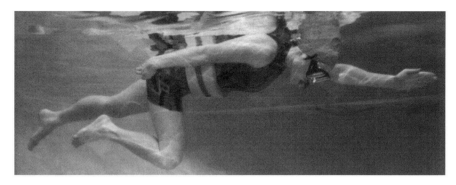

Figure 4-24. Quadruped level III. (Courtesy of AquaTechnics Consulting Group, Inc., Aptos, CA.)

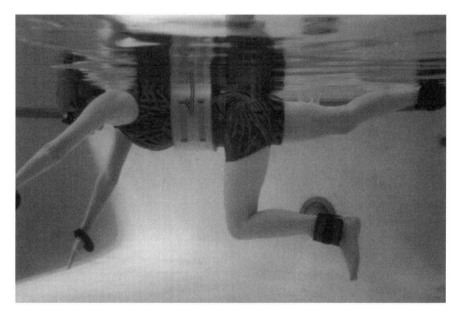

Figure 4-25. Quadruped level IV. (Courtesy of AquaTechnics Consulting Group, Inc., Aptos, CA.)

- Level I: The therapist instructs the patient to float in a prone position, with the knees flexed to 25 degrees and the arms at 0-degree flexion (Figure 4-26). The cervical spine is maintained at approximately 20 degrees of flexion. Proper breathing and relaxation are emphasized. Upper extremity movement of the entire shoulder complex begins with small, rotatory movement of the lower arms under the chest, as if the patient is rototilling water. The hips are maintained at 25-degree flexion. Small flexion-extension knee movements are initiated simultaneously with small, rotatory arm movements. Both movements cause propulsion. A lateral rocking movement is taught so that the patient "log-rolls" in the water. This motion minimizes the amount of segmental stress placed across each motion segment in the lumbar spine. The patient performs the exercise pattern

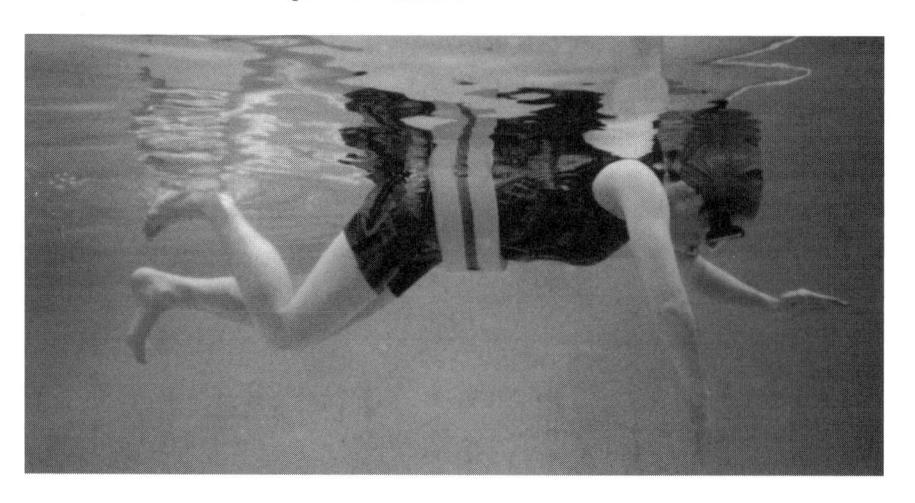

Figure 4-26. Log-roll swim level I. (Courtesy of AquaTechnics Consulting Group, Inc., Aptos, CA.)

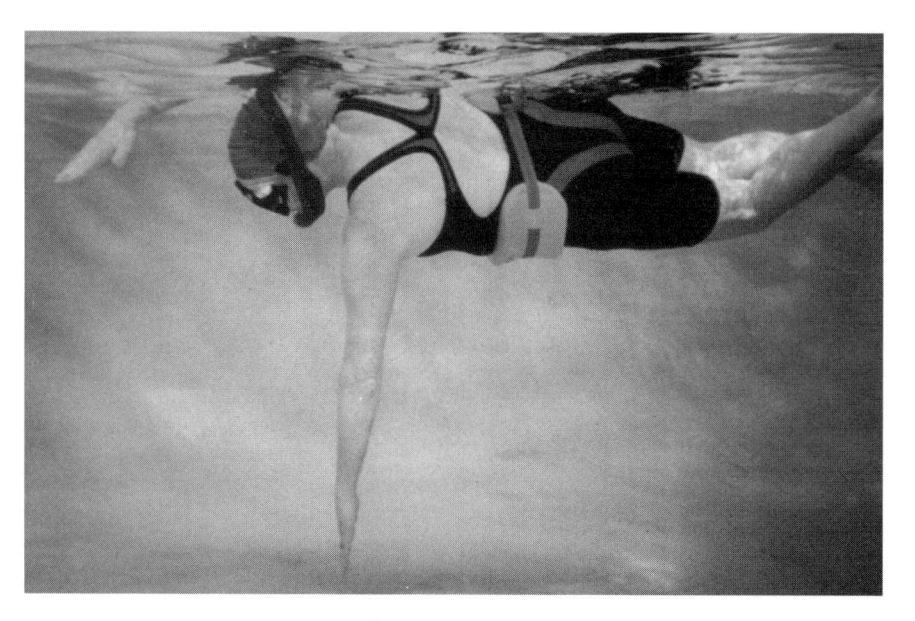

Figure 4-27. Log-roll swim level II. (Courtesy of AquaTechnics Consulting Group, Inc., Aptos, CA.)

for 5 minutes at 50% of maximum velocity. Lateral flexion and rotation must be avoided.

- Level II: Level II begins with the upper extremities performing scooping movements under the body (Figure 4-27). Each arm is lifted in an arc for recovery above the head just like the freestyle stroke, and the hand enters the water to repeat the cycle. The log-roll pattern must be maintained. When upper body motion is correctly performed, level I kicking is added. This exercise continues for 5 minutes at 50% of maximum velocity.

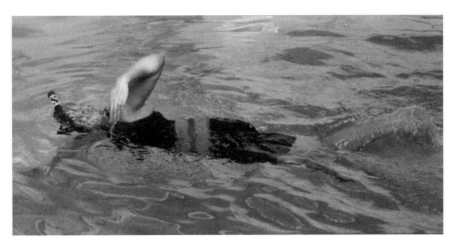

Figure 4-28. Log-roll swim level III. (Courtesy of AquaTechnics Consulting Group, Inc., Aptos, CA.)

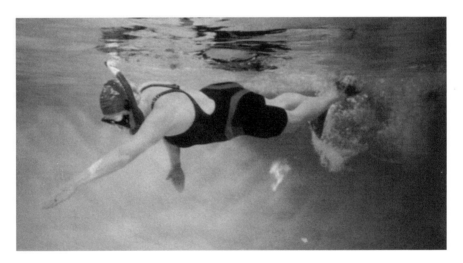

Figure 4-29. Log-roll swim level IV. (Courtesy of AquaTechnics Consulting Group, Inc., Aptos, CA.)

- Level III: The level II exercise continues, but the arm motion advances to normal freestyle, and kicking begins from the hip rather than the knee (Figure 4-28). This pattern continues for 5 minutes at 50% of maximum potential velocity.
- Level IV: Level IV is similar to level III, but the flotation belt is eliminated and short-blade fins are added (Figure 4-29). This pattern continues for 10 minutes at 80% of maximum potential velocity.

At this point, the patient can eliminate the mask, snorkel, and fins and can begin a spine-stabilized swimming program.

Table 4-3. Swimming Stroke Phases (Freestyle)

   I. Entry phase
    A. Hand entry
    B. Hand submersion (ride)
  II. Pull phase
    A. Insweep
    B. Outsweep
    C. Finish
 III. Recovery phase
    A. Exit
    B. Arm swing

Source: AquaTechnics Consulting Group, Inc., Aptos, CA.

SPINE-STABILIZED SWIMMING PROGRAMS

Once a patient's stabilization skills have progressed to the point at which swimming is possible, a thorough analysis of stroke technique and its effect on spine motion is critical [43]. The following overview focuses on lumbar spine injury and indicates the role that the cervical spine plays in the mechanics of lumbar aquatic motion.

Analysis of stroke mechanics, like gait analysis, should be done in an ordered, sequential manner so that all deficits and their relationships are carefully and fully scrutinized. Typically, we begin the analysis at the head and work distally.

Prone Swimming

In prone swimming, the patient's head should be midline. Breathing should occur by turning the head, that is, by rotating the head along the axial plane. There should be no craning (suboccipital cervical extension and rotation) or cervical extension and rotation (C2–C7) (see Figure 4-2). Body roll also contributes to proper breathing mechanics and is essential to minimize dysfunctional cervical positioning and subsequent pain. The cervical spine should be kept in the neutral position along the sagittal plane because excessive extension causes the legs and torso to drop in the water, and excessive flexion can cause a struggle for air [2,3,11,18,43].

The upper-body arm position is evaluated by stroke phase (Table 4-3). Freestyle is made up of three phases. The entry phase includes hand entry and hand submersion (*ride*). The pull phase incorporates insweep, outsweep, and finish components. The recovery phase includes the exit and arm swing [41]. Several stroke defects can cause poor lumbar mechanics. If the arm abducts beyond 180 degrees, lateral lumbar flexion and rotation occurs (Figure 4-30). During the pull phase, decreased body rotation can cause lateral lumbar flexion and rotation that stress the lumbar motion segments, particularly the annular fibers surrounding the nucleus pulposus. Inadequate strength in the triceps during the finish phase results in low arm recovery, which in turn generates secondary lateral flexion and rotation through the lumbar spine. During recovery, inadequate body roll causes the neck to crane, which results in a struggle for air and accompanying lateral flexion and rotation through the lumbar spine [2,3,8,11,18,43].

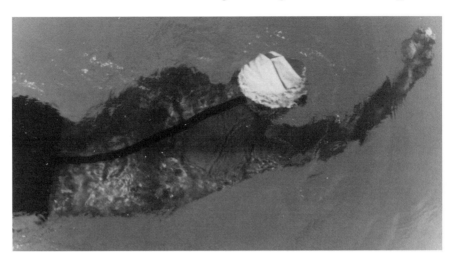

Figure 4-30. This swimmer's arm abducts beyond 180 degrees during the entry phase of freestyle. This stroke defect creates lateral lumbar flexion (*line*) and lumbar segmental rotation. (Courtesy of AquaTechnics Consulting Group, Inc., Aptos, CA.)

Trunk motion is monitored closely for any primary or secondary lumbar flexion, both sagittal and coronal, or for axial rotation. If flexion and rotation are not corrected by simple changes in stroke mechanics, additional proprioceptive cues can be provided by taping the lumbar spine region. The tape pulls on the skin each time the lumbar spine moves in a segmental manner, that is, when the patient generates excessive lumbar rotation or lateral lumbar flexion [19] (Figure 4-31). Table 4-4 delineates how these and other primary peripheral joint freestyle stroke defects and secondary effects can create abnormal spine mechanics during swimming and cause or exacerbate a painful spine dysfunction.

Flip turns are discouraged. Instead, the patient uses a stabilized turn in which a vertical position is reached before turning. This vertical position allows the patient to stabilize the spine when preparing to change direction. Eventually, a horizontal spin is incorporated into the turn, and the vertical position is eliminated. Flip turns may then be resumed [2,11,18,25].

Supine Swimming

It is best to start with a simple kicking program, with the patient in the supine position and arms at the side, because adequate stabilization can be maintained easily. The use of fins is often suggested to improve propulsion. In the supine position, extension of the cervical spine induces lumbar extension. In contrast, cervical flexion causes the patient to "sit" in the water, with lowered leg position and decreased propulsion. Extreme cervical extension or flexion is avoided in favor of a more neutral, stabilized cervical posture [2,3,11,18,43].

Problems with stroke technique usually can be solved with simple changes in stroke mechanics or by adding adaptive equipment. For example, struggling for air can be resolved by the addition of a mask and snorkel. Trunk position can be

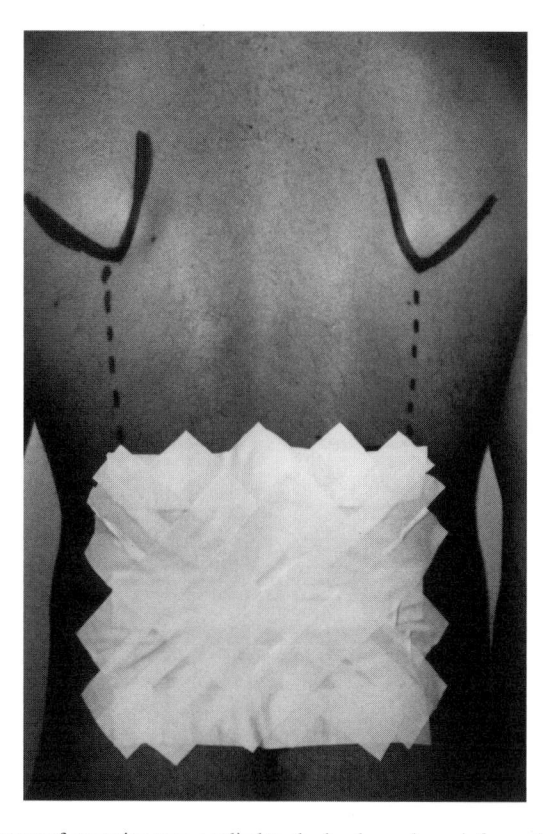

Figure 4-31. Waterproof strapping tape applied to the lumbar spine reinforces lumbar proprioceptive awareness and helps to minimize lumbar rotation and lateral flexion. (Courtesy of AquaTechnics Consulting Group, Inc., Aptos, CA.)

improved by using the taping technique already described. Poor propulsion can be remedied by appropriate fins. Hand paddles can provide better kinesthetic awareness of hand and arm position [2,11,18].

SPINAL PAIN IN SWIMMERS

Repetitive microtrauma from swimming is a primary cause of spinal injury. If the average competitive swimmer swims 5,000 yd freestyle per day, 5 days each week, using 15 strokes per pool length, and breathes every other stroke, he or she performs approximately 600,000 arm movements, 300,000 cervical spine rotations, and 600,000 lumbar rotatory movements per year. Supplementary land-based flexibility and strength programs without attention to proper spinal mechanics can cause or contribute to spine injury and pain [5]. Mutoh et al. [44] retrospectively studied 66 elite Japanese aquatic athletes, including competitive swimmers, divers, water polo players, and synchronized swimmers. The lower back was the most common site of injury for all four groups; 37.1% of the 19 competitive swimmers had chronic low-back pain. This finding is similar to Mutoh's 1983 study, in which 33% of the 51 Japanese swimmers he studied had low-back pain [45]. Mutoh's findings are in con-

Table 4-4. Freestyle Stroke Defects

Primary Peripheral Joint Stroke Defect	Secondary Effect	Spine Reaction
Head high	Lower body sinks	Increased cervical extension
		Increased lumbar extension
Head low	Upper body sinks	Increased lumbar flexion
Crane breathing	Lower body sinks	Increased cervical and suboccipital extension
	Contralateral shoulder sinks	Increased cervical rotation
		Increased lumbar lateral flexion and rotation
Crossover hand entry	Lateral body movement	Increased lumbar lateral flexion and rotation
Wide hand entry	Contralateral shoulder roll	Increased cervical rotation
		Increased lumbar lateral flexion and rotation
Inefficient pull power	Upper body sinks	Increased cervical rotation
	Difficulty breathing	Increased cervical extension
		Increased lumbar extension
		Increased lumbar lateral flexion and rotation
Increased hip flexion	Decreased kick propulsion	Increased cervical extension
	Lower body sinks	Increased lumbar extension
		Increased lumbar lateral flexion and rotation
Crossover kick	Decreased kick propulsion	Increased cervical extension
	Increased hip roll	Increased lumbar extension
	Lower body sinks	Increased compensatory lumbar lateral flexion and rotation
Increased knee flexion	Decreased kick propulsion	Increased cervical extension
	Lower body sinks	Increased lumbar extension
Increased ankle dorsiflexion	Decreased kick propulsion	Increased cervical extension
	Increased hip roll	Increased lumbar extension
	Lower body sinks	Increased compensatory lumbar lateral flexion and rotation

Source: AquaTechnics Consulting Group, Inc., Aptos, CA.

tradistinction to a 1980 study in which shoulder pain was the most common orthopedic problem in competitive swimming [46]. Although all spinal structures are presumably at risk during swimming activities, the biomechanics of certain strokes predispose particular structures to increased risk.

Biomechanics of Spinal Injury in Swimmers

Of the four competitive strokes, freestyle and backstroke most increase lumbar segmental axial rotation and torque force, thereby placing the annulus fibrosus in particular jeopardy [47–50]. In elite swimmers, this risk factor would seem to decrease in importance because of improved stroke technique. Although they are trained to roll their bodies as a unit (nonsegmentally) [2,8,11,51,52], thus minimizing torque force across individual lumbar motion segments and also decreasing head drag forces, elite swimmers probably subject these segments to greater force per stroke. Paradoxically, they increase the chance of injury due to repetitive microtrauma [43,47,53–57] (S Kenney, personal communication, 1991). Risk of lumbar facet pain increases with strokes such as the butterfly and breaststroke, which include an accentuated lumbar extension (Figure 4-32) [52]. When performing these strokes, elite

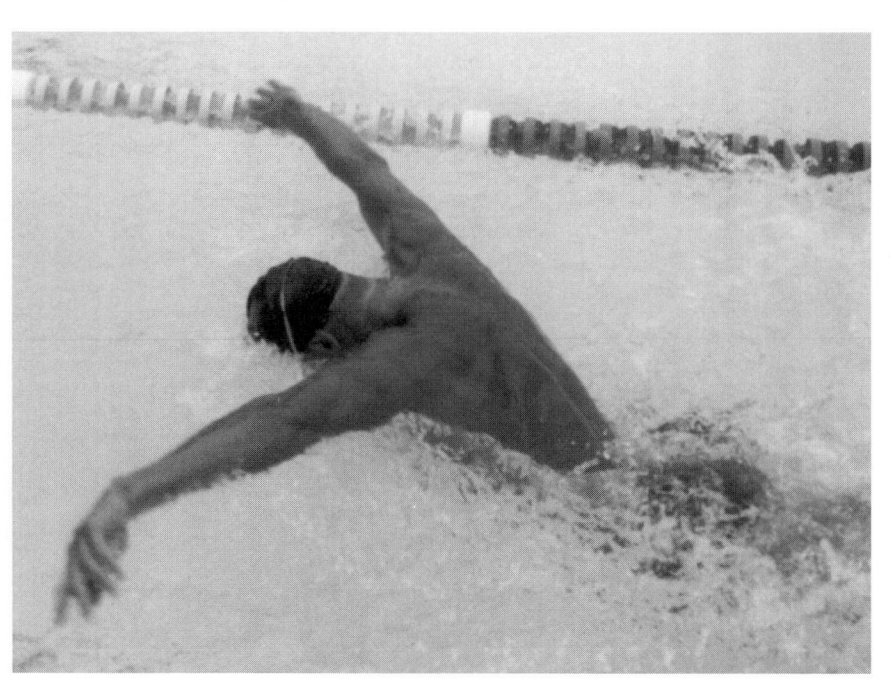

Figure 4-32. The risk of lumbar facet pain increases with strokes that include an accentuated lumbar extension, such as the butterfly. (Courtesy of AquaTechnics Consulting Group, Inc., Aptos, CA.)

athletes, in particular, are at risk due to an exaggerated undulation that increases sagittal motion (i.e., extension and flexion). This undulation compounds the risk of facet injury due to repetitive microtrauma. Even with the breaststroke, traditionally a controlled swimming style, recent advances in stroke technique have resulted in a significant increase in sagittal plane motion by emphasizing undulatory rather than linear, plane horizontal motion (S Kenney, personal communication, 1991). Although injury to the pars interarticularis may be seen more frequently in competitive divers [54], many swimmers with a quiescent spondylolysis may become symptomatic due to the repetitive extensions that occur with breaststroke, butterfly, starts, and turns. Furthermore, the risk of developing spondylolysis due to stress placed by these strokes on the posterior column of the spine remains unclear.

Although injuries to the thoracic spine seem to occur less frequently and appear to be more easily rehabilitated, these structures are nonetheless at risk. Most commonly seen is thoracic facet pain, especially with strokes that generate a great degree of increased segmental rotatory motion at particular thoracic motion segments, such as freestyle and backstroke. The extension required in butterfly and breaststroke may cause facet joint dysfunction and pain. The pain, which may be caused by inflammation, results from repetitive facet compression, distraction, and shear forces [3,8,11]. We believe that during the pull phase, compressive forces are generated by the ipsilateral latissimus dorsi, scapular retractors, and long thoracic spinal extensor muscle groups. Ipsilateral thoracic spinal muscle groups produce an extension to counter the flexion of the latissimus dorsi. The contralateral thoracic spinal muscle groups stabilize the thoracic spine, pre-

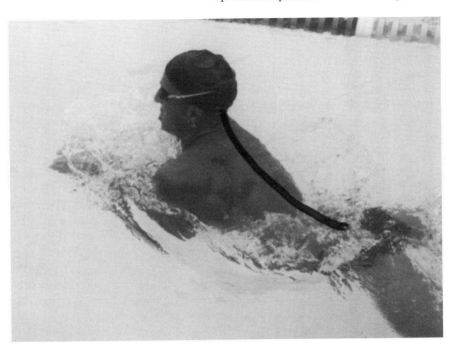

Figure 4-33. Breaststroke requires repetitive end-range cervical extension (*line*) for breathing. This increases the risk of cervical posterior element injury that can produce facet pain. (Courtesy of AquaTechnics Consulting Group, Inc., Aptos, CA.)

venting untoward lateral flexion toward the pull-phase side. Passive distractive forces affect the ipsilateral facet during the recovery phase due to activation of the ipsilateral scapular protractors, relaxation of the scapular retractors, inactivation of latissimus dorsi, and relative relaxation of the thoracic spinal extensor muscle groups [9,18,51,55,56].

Thoracic costovertebral joints may be injured as a result of significantly increased vital capacity and enhanced motion of the chest wall and ribs. These joints may be compromised further by arm elevation and the consequent increase of tension on the rib system. Additionally, faulty stroke mechanics resulting in increased rotation through the thoracic spine may contribute to costovertebral joint pain [18,51].

The cervical spine is subjected continuously to repetitive microtrauma from the mechanics of breathing. Annular as well as facet injuries are most commonly seen with freestyle stroke because of the significant rotation required for side breathing [3,18,51]. Occasionally, a side-breathing technique is used during the butterfly, also placing the cervical segments at increased risk. Extension, which is seen with breaststroke and butterfly (Figure 4-33), increases the chance of cervical posterior element injury, resulting in cervical facet pain. Cervical extension can also increase intradiscal pressure, compromising the intervertebral disc [57]. Although the backstroke requires little rotation for breathing, exceptional stabilization of the cervical segments in a relatively neutral position is needed to reduce drag forces. As a result, fewer intrinsic cervical segmental injuries tend to occur from this stroke, but muscular strain to the cervical dynamic stabilizing soft tissues, such as the paraspinal muscle groups, is common. There is significant risk of catastrophic cervical spine injury caused by impact loading [58–61]. The greatest potential for this type of injury is found in faulty start mechanics and, less commonly, with impact loading of the cervical spine during a missed turn, particularly during the backstroke, in which the swimmer cannot see the oncoming wall or may fail to observe overhead warning flags [18,51].

Patients with Scheuermann's kyphosis were found to develop increased pain during swimming, particularly during the butterfly stroke, in a study by Wilson and Lindseth [62]. Of the four competitive strokes, the butterfly includes the greatest end-range extension of the diseased, less mobile thoracic motion segments. Increased pectoral and associated chest and abdominal muscle contractions during the pull phase of a butterfly stroke may cause compressive forces that further damage anterior column structures [63]. Because these muscles are also significantly active during the pull phase of the freestyle and breaststroke [27,28,55,56,64], repetitive end-range extension microtrauma may be the primary biomechanical source of pain in the butterfly. Although kyphotic patients can be managed conservatively with daily bracing, additional time out of their braces was suggested to allow continued swimming. When the butterfly was avoided, no deleterious change was noted [62]. Additionally, because of the swimmer's horizontal position in the water and the buoyant effect of the water, the axial compressive forces on the spine [27] are reduced significantly. This positioning and buoyancy may significantly mitigate mechanical risk factors that may cause this condition to progress.

The prevalence of adolescent idiopathic scoliosis is approximately 2–3% [65]. In the athletic population, the average frequency of idiopathic scoliosis has been reported to be 2% [29], and the incidence of functional scoliosis, 33.5% [66]. The higher incidence of functional scoliosis in the athletic population may be due to larger unilateral torque forces developed in particular activities, such as serving and throwing [29]. More recent work by Becker [67] (personal communication, 1991), who screened 336 swimmers at the Junior Olympic Swimming Championships, East, 1983, showed an incidence of 6.9% idiopathic scoliosis and 16% functional scoliosis. The 6.9% figure is roughly three times the reported incidence of structural idiopathic scoliosis, but the 16% figure is below the incidence reported by Krahl and Steinbruck [66]. One hundred percent of the functional curves, however, were toward the dominant-hand side, which, according to Yeater, consistently produces greater pull-phase peak forces than the nondominant side [65]. Further studies summarized by Becker revealed histologic and morphologic changes in the paraspinal and gluteus muscles, secondary adaptation of supporting vertebral soft tissues, and adaptive changes in muscles to meet specific repetitive functional demands [67]. However, if curve progression is truly facilitated by the asymmetric functional demands that swimming places on the spine, then a therapeutic exercise program could theoretically be designed to counter them. Moreover, exercise alone is unable to inhibit the progression of a scoliotic curve [67], and it remains to be shown whether exercise can accelerate curve progression. Additionally, the most recent advances in swimming techniques, especially in the freestyle, emphasize symmetric motion (e.g., alternate-side breathing) and minimize repetitive unilateral torsion and lateral flexion. Proper coaching should help to further de-emphasize the potential effect of a stronger, dominant side on the spine. We believe that swimming is not contraindicated for adolescents with functional or idiopathic scoliosis. We recommend appropriate training by the patients' therapists and coaches, who should know swimming technique and mechanics. In fact, with proper technique, aquatic activity may help scoliotic patients.

CONCLUSION

Repetitive microtrauma from aquatic rehabilitation, as well as the land-based flexibility and strength programs that are performed without attention to proper spinal mechanics, can cause or contribute to spinal injury and pain. Because the spinal axis is essentially a force transmitter for peripheral joint motion, both direct spinal injury and altered biomechanics at sites distant from the spine can change spinal mechanics and cause dysfunction and pain. A series of aquatic stabilization exercises has been designed that incorporates the intrinsic properties of water and enhances rehabilitative efforts. When these exercises are mastered, injured patients can soon advance to spine-safe swimming or other high-level aquatic training activities [68]. Swimming programs, in particular, require that close attention be paid to proper swim-stroke biomechanics and to the effect that abnormal mechanics may have on the spine. This attention ensures the most rapid rehabilitation of painful spinal disorders.

Acknowledgments

The authors would like to thank Carolinda E. Hill (Scientific Publications Office, Baylor Research Institute, Dallas, TX) for reading and editing the manuscript; Diane Rothhammer-Sheets for the use of equipment; Rod Fleming, P.T., and Murray Fleming, P.T., for the use of their swimming pool; and Shenay Moschetti and Allison Miller for their photographic assistance.

REFERENCES

1. Canadian Olympic Association. Canadian Olympic Association Report. Canada; Autumn 1982.
2. Cole AJ, Moschetti ML, Eagleston RA. Getting backs in the swim. Rehabil Manage 1992;5:62.
3. Cole AJ, Farrell JP, Stratton SA. Cervical Spine Athletic Injuries: A Pain in the Neck. In J Press (ed), Physical Medicine and Rehabilitation Clinics of North America. Philadelphia: Saunders, 1994;37.
4. Press JM, Herring SA, Kibler WB (eds). Rehabilitation of Musculoskeletal Disorders. The Textbook of Military Medicine. Borden Institute, Office of the Surgeon General (in press).
5. Kibler WB, Chandler TJ, Pace BK. Principles of Rehabilitation After Chronic Tendon Injuries. In AFH Renstrom, WB Leadbetter (eds), Clinics in Sports Medicine. Philadelphia: Saunders, 1992;661.
6. Herring SA. Rehabilitation of muscle injuries. Med Sci Sports Exerc 1990;22:453.
7. Paris S. The Spine and Swimming. In S Hockschuler (ed), Spine: State of the Art Reviews. Philadelphia: Hanley & Belfus, 1990;351.
8. Cole AJ, Herring SA. The Role of the Physiatrist in the Management of Lumbar Spine Pain. In DC Tollison (ed), The Handbook of Pain Management (2nd ed). Baltimore: Williams & Wilkins, 1994;85.
9. Scovazzo M, Browne A, Pink M, et al. The painful shoulder during freestyle swimming: an electromyographic cinematographic analysis of twelve muscles. Am J Sports Med 1991;19:577.
10. Cole AJ, Reid M. Clinical assessment of the shoulder. J Back Musculoskel Rehabil 1992;2:7.
11. Cole AJ, Moschetti ML, Eagleston RA. Lumbar Spine Aquatic Rehabilitation: A Sports Medicine Approach. In DC Tollison (ed), The Handbook of Pain Management (2nd ed). Baltimore: Williams & Wilkins, 1994;386.
12. Kadaba MP, Cole AJ. Intramuscular wire electromyography of the subscapularis. J Orthop Res 1992;10:394.

13. Wilder RP, Sobel J, Cole AJ, et al. Overuse injuries of the hip and pelvis in sports. J Back Musculoskel Rehabil 1994;4:236.

14. Kibler WB. Clinical aspects of muscle injury. Med Sci Sports Exerc 1990;22:450.

15. Saal J. Rehabilitation of the Injured Athlete. In J DeLisa (ed), Rehabilitation Medicine: Principles and Practice. Philadelphia: Lippincott, 1988;840.

16. Saal JA, Saal JS. Later Stage Management of Lumbar Spine Problems. In S Herring (ed), Physical Medicine and Rehabilitation Clinics of North America. Philadelphia: Saunders, 1991;205.

17. Saal JA. Dynamic muscular stabilization in the nonoperative treatment of lumbar pain syndromes. Orthop Rev 1990;19:691.

18. Cole AJ, Campbell DR, Berson D, et al. Swimming. In RG Watkins (ed), The Spine in Sports. St. Louis: Mosby, 1996;362.

19. Cole A, Eagleston R, Moschetti ML, et al. Lumbar torque: a new proprioceptive approach. Poster presented at the Annual Meeting of the North American Spine Society, Keystone, CO; August 1–3, 1991.

20. Minor MA, Hewett JE, Webel RR, et al. Efficacy of physical conditioning exercise in patients with rheumatoid arthritis and osteoarthritis. Arthritis Rheum 1989;32:1396.

21. Goldstein E, Simkin A, Epstein L, Peritz E. The influence of weight-bearing water exercises on bone density of post-menopausal women. Unpublished results, Zinman College of Physical Education, Jerusalem, 1995.

22. LeFort SM, Hannah TE. Return to work following an aquafitness and muscle strengthening program for the low back injured. Arch Phys Med Rehabil 1994;75:1247.

23. Cole AJ. When to call for help. J Phys Ed Recreation Dance 1993;(Jan):55.

24. Reister VC, Cole AJ. Start active, stay active in the water. J Phys Ed Recreation Dance 1993;(Jan):52.

25. Cole AJ, Moschetti ML, Eagleston RA. Swimming. In AH White (ed), Spine Care. St. Louis: Mosby, 1995;727.

26. Cole AJ, Moschetti ML, Eagleston RA. The water scale: a classification system for aquatic exercise. Manuscript in preparation, 1997.

27. Miller F. Fluids. In College Physics (4th ed). New York: Harcourt, Brace, Jovanovich, 1977;271.

28. Piette G, Clarys JP. Telemetric EMG of the Front Crawl Movement. In J Terauds, W Bedingfield (eds), Swimming III. Baltimore, MD: University Park Press, 1979;153.

29. Kuprian W. Physical Therapy for Sports. Philadelphia: Saunders, 1982;377.

30. Councilman J. The Science of Swimming. Englewood Cliffs, NJ: Prentice Hall, 1968.

31. Martin R. Swimming: Forces on Aquatic Animals and Humans. In CL Vaughan (ed), Biomechanics of Sport. Boca Raton, FL: CRC Press, 1989;35.

32. Costill D, Cahill P, Eddy D. Metabolic responses to submaximal exercise in three water temperatures. J Appl Physiol 1967;22:628.

33. Kirby RL, Sacamano JT, Balch DE, Kriellaars OJ. Oxygen consumption during exercise in a heated pool. Arch Phys Med Rehabil 1984;65:21.

34. Kolb M. Principles of underwater exercise. Phys Ther Rev 1957;37:361.

35. Kreighbaum E, Barthels K. Biomechanics: A Qualitative Approach for Studying Human Movement (2nd ed). Minneapolis: Burgess, 1985;421.

36. Martin WH III, Montgomery J, Snell PG, et al. Cardiovascular adaptations to intense swim training in sedentary middle-aged men and women. Circulation 1987;75:323.

37. McArdle W, Katch F, Katch V. Energy Expenditure During Walking, Jogging, Running, and Swimming. In W McArdle, F Katch, V Katch (eds), Exercise Physiology: Energy, Nutrition, and Human Performance. Philadelphia: Lea & Febiger, 1986;158.

38. Panjabi M, Abumi K, Duranceau J, Oxland T. Spinal stability and intersegmental muscle forces. A biomechanical model. Spine 1989;14:194.

39. Shirazi-Adl A, Ahmed A, Shrivastava S. Mechanical response of a lumbar motion segment in axial torque alone and combined with compression. Spine 1989;11:914.

40. Constant F, Collin JF, Guillemin F, Boulangé M. Effectiveness of spa therapy in chronic low back pain: a randomized clinical trial. J Rheumatol 1995;22:1315.

41. Eagleston R. Aquatic stabilization programs. Presented at the Conference on Aggressive Non-surgical Rehabilitation and Lumbar Spine and Sports Injuries, San Francisco Spine Institute. San Francisco, CA: March 23, 1989.

42. Brewster NT, Howie CR. That sinking feeling. BMJ 1992;305:1579.

43. Maglisco E. Swimming Even Faster. Sunnyvale, CA: Mayfield, 1993.

44. Mutoh Y, Miwako T, Mitsumasa M. Chronic Injuries of Elite Competitive Swimmers, Divers, Water Polo Players, and Synchronized Swimmers. In VB Ungerecht, K Wilke (eds), Swimming Science. Champaign, IL: Human Kinetics Books, 1988;333.

45. Mutoh Y. Mechanism and prevention of swimming injury. Jpn J Sports Science 1983;2:527.

46. Richardson A, Jobe F, Collins H. The shoulder in competitive swimming. Am J Sports Med 1980;8:159.

47. Bogduk N, Twomey LT. Clinical Anatomy of the Lumbar Spine (2nd ed). New York: Churchill Livingstone, 1991.

48. Farfan H. Effects of torsion on the intervertebral joints. Can J Surg 1969;12:336.

49. Farfan HF, Cossette JW, Robertson GH, et al. The effects of torsion on the lumbar intervertebral joints: the role of torsion in the production of disc degeneration. J Bone Joint Surg [Am] 1970;52:468.

50. Goldstein JD, Berger PE, Windler GE, Jackson DW. Spine injuries in gymnasts and swimmers: an epidemiologic investigation. Am J Sports Med 1991;19:463.

51. Cole AJ, Moschetti ML, Eagleston RA. Spine pain: aquatic rehabilitation strategies. J Back Musculoskel Rehabil 1994;4:273.

52. Ruoti R, Morris D, Cole AJ. Aquatic Rehabilitation. Philadelphia: Lippincott, 1997.

53. Rucker K, Cole AJ, Weinstein S. Lumbar Spine Pain: A Clinical Approach. Philadelphia: Andover Medical Publishers (accepted for publication in 1995).

54. Rossi R. Spondylolysis, spondylolisthesis and sports. J Sports Med Phys Fitness 1978;18:317.

55. Nuber GW, Jobe FW, Perry J, et al. Fine wire electromyography analysis of muscles of the shoulder during swimming. Am J Sports Med 1986;14:7.

56. Pink M, Perry J, Browne A, et al. The normal shoulder during freestyle swimming: an electromyographic and cinematographic analysis of twelve muscles. Am J Sports Med 1991;19:569.

57. White A. Clinical anatomy and biomechanics. Presented at the meeting of the Cervical Spine and Upper Extremity in Sports and Industry, San Francisco Spine Institute. San Francisco, CA: April 1, 1990.

58. Bailes JE, Herman JM, Quigley MR, et al. Diving injuries of the cervical spine. Surg Neurol 1990;34:155.

59. Good R, Nickel V. Cervical spine injuries resulting from water sports. Spine 1980;5:502.

60. Kewalramani L, Taylor R. Injuries to the cervical spine from diving accidents. J Trauma 1975;15:130.

61. Kiwerski J. Cervical spine injuries caused by diving into water. Paraplegia 1980;18:101.

62. Wilson F, Lindseth R. The adolescent swimmer's back. Am J Sports Med 1982;10:174.

63. Benson D, Wolf A, Shoji H. Can the Milwaukee brace patient participate in competitive athletics? Am J Sports Med 1977;5:7.

64. Clarys JP, Piette G. A Review of EMG in Swimming: Explanation of Facts and/or Feedback Information. In AP Hollander, PA Huijing, G deGroot (eds), Biomechanics and Medicine in Swimming. Champaign, IL: Human Kinetics Books, 1983;153.

65. Yeater RA, Martin RB, White MK, Gilson KH. Tethered swimming forces in the crawl, breast, and back strokes and their relationship to competitive performance. J Biomech 1981;14:527.

66. Krahl H, Steinbruck K. Sportsachaden and Sportverletzungen. der Wirbelsaule Arztebl 1978;19.

67. Becker TJ. Scoliosis in Swimmers. In JV Ciullo (ed), Clinics in Sports Medicine. Philadelphia: Saunders, 1986;149.

68. Wilder RP, Brennan D, Schotte DE. A standard measure for exercise prescription for aqua running. Am J Sports Med 1993;21:45.

5

Hydrotherapeutic Applications in Arthritis Rehabilitation

Gwendolyn Garrett

It is believed that early humans discovered thermal springs by tracking wounded animals, who instinctively knew the healing benefits of warm water immersion. Medical doctrines of the Greeks and Romans reveal the widespread usage of water immersion for medicinal purposes for a variety of ills, including arthritis. Observations have been made through history that immersion in thermal mineral waters resulted in shrinking of peripheral edema, reduction of joint pain, and improvement in joint mobility. Hydrotherapy combined with heat is among the oldest rehabilitative treatments for arthritis [1]. Today, passive and active treatments in a warm-water environment play a significant and distinct role in the rehabilitation of arthritis.

The rheumatic diseases affect the joints, muscles, and connective tissues of the body and appear to be a result of a complex of interacting mechanical, biological, biochemical, and enzymatic feedback loops [2]. The word *arthritis* literally means joint inflammation. The precise mechanisms causing these structures to be attacked are incompletely understood and, in some instances, seem to be triggered by a preceding infectious process, in others by a sudden autoimmune response, and in some cases perhaps as a response to joint stress. There is considerable individual variation in symptom magnitude, joint involvement, and disease duration. A symptom complex of joint swelling, pain, stiffness, inflammation, and limitation of range of motion (ROM) is typically produced, irrespective of cause [3]. The most prevalent forms of the disease are osteoarthritis, a degenerative joint disease in which one or many joints undergo degenerative changes, including loss of articular cartilage and the formation of osteophytes, and rheumatoid arthritis, an autoimmune disease that produces both acute inflammatory and progressive joint damage [4–5]. In the case of osteoarthritis, age is the most significant risk factor, but as with many other forms of arthritis, the condition may result from anatomic or metabolic predisposition. More commonly, the pathogenesis is simply unknown [6]. There are thought to be more than 100 types of arthritis, including ankylosing spondylitis, fibromyalgia, lupus, and juvenile rheumatoid arthritis [7]. Most of these are chronic conditions for which there is no definitive cure but a series of medical management options. Left untreated, many are progressive, and can cause significant impairment, disability, and handicap over time. For the great majority of arthritides, medical management can be very helpful in controlling symptom magnitude, limiting progression of the disease, and reducing disability. The typical approach is (1) to control the underlying disease and reduce symptoms, (2) to preserve and maintain function through activity modulation and adaptation, and (3) to prevent disability through activity regulation, joint protection, and lifestyle adjustment.

DEMOGRAPHICS OF ARTHRITIS

Arthritis is the number one cause of disability and the most common clinical complaint in the United States [8]. Recent estimates are that by the year 2020, 59.4 million Americans (18.2% of the country's population) will have some form of arthritis; the current prevalence is 15% [9]. The same studies show that nearly 3% of the population is functionally limited by their arthritis. More alarming, in 1994, Guccione stated that 60 million adults in the United States were thought to have some form of osteoarthritis, an estimate much higher than the Arthritis Foundation has suggested [10]. As the general population ages, the numbers will continue to rise. Overall, women are more commonly afflicted than men; of the 40 million who suffer today, 23 million are female [2]. Arthritis strikes children and those in their twenties and thirties, and it is almost universal by age 70.

The direct and indirect costs of arthritis are great. Considering that one in every six Americans is affected, billions are spent annually on physician costs, radiology and lab fees, hospitalization, surgery, therapy, medication, and medical equipment. In 1994 alone, medical care associated with arthritis cost $54.6 billion [9]. Despite advanced technology and current research efforts, arthritis still accounts for 427 million days of lost work annually and is the leading cause of industrial absenteeism in the United States [8].

DISEASE EFFECTS

The rheumatic diseases share common signs and symptoms: pain, general stiffness, joint inflammation, swelling, and diminished ROM [11]. The primary impairments associated with arthritis are the alterations of normal structures and functions of bones, muscles, and joints of the musculoskeletal system. Deformities and loss of function in arthritis are caused by changes in articular and periarticular tissues directly or indirectly related to the disease process. Early tissue changes cause pain and stiffness that interfere with movement before there is actual loss of function [12]. Muscles and joints tend to become stiff, tense, and weak. Tense muscles press on nerve endings, also making movements painful and difficult. Persistent pain causes restricted joint motion and inhibition of muscle contraction, which results in further loss of joint mobility and disuse atrophy of adjacent muscle groups. This leads to a weakening of the muscles essential to joint protection and a vicious cycle of lack of activity and loss of function. Inactivity causes substantial weakness and loss of tissue from all elements of the musculoskeletal system. Deficits such as poor endurance and fatigue associated with aerobic deconditioning are viewed as reversible functional losses for the arthritic patient.

The weakness associated with arthritis may have multiple origins. Joint effusion has been shown to decrease active strength across the joint [13]. Strength may be

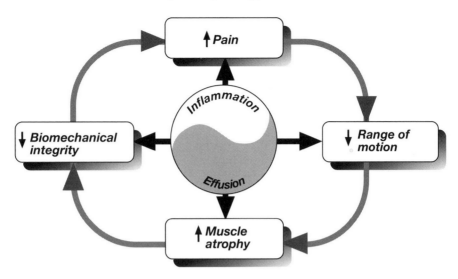

Figure 5-1. Cycle of arthritic dysfunction. (Adapted from JE Hicks. Exercise for patients with inflammatory arthritis. J Musculoskel Med 1989;10:40.)

reduced because of decreased biomechanical integrity, with consequent reflex inhibition of the joint effector muscles [14]. Pain-induced inactivity leads to deconditioning and atrophy [14]. The medical management of arthritis may involve medications that create muscle atrophy, such as corticosteroids, even on low-dose regimens [15]. The arthritic process may involve muscle directly, producing an inflammatory myopathy and consequent diminished strength [16]. Other causes have also been found to cause muscle weakness, including nerve involvement, muscle fiber–type alteration, and cellular metabolic process changes. Figure 5-1 demonstrates the vicious cycle that an active arthritic process can develop. These changes include loss of bone, muscle, and connective tissue; a reduction in joint ROM, muscle strength, and endurance; and a marked decline in fitness [17]. Prolonged inactivity results in loss of flexibility and physical capacity, deconditioning, and deterioration of functional abilities, such as reaching overhead, dressing, getting up from the toilet, and walking.

As limiting as the loss of physical functioning may be, arthritis also affects other, nonphysical aspect of a person's life: the way he or she feels about himself or herself and others and how he or she works, sleeps, eats, and relaxes [18]. These changes in lifestyle can lead to depression; social isolation; and an inability to fulfill social, family, and societal roles. Through proper treatment, however, symptoms and disease progression can often be managed or diminished.

EXERCISE IN ARTHRITIS

Many believe that exercise and rest are the cornerstone of the overall medical management of arthritic diseases. The incorporation of exercise as an essential part of the management of patients with arthritis dates at least to Roman times. Although exercise may or may not change the progression of the underlying rheumatic process in a given individual, it can play an invaluable role in keeping muscle strength and joint ROM as normal as possible without further damaging diseased intra- and extra-articular tissues, aiding contracture prevention, slowing down other deformities, and preventing much of the loss of function [19]. Specific goals of exercise for these populations include maintaining strength and endurance, preserving joint motion, retaining the ability to perform activities of daily living, preserving bone density, and reducing pain [20].

Beals said, "Rheumatoid patients as a group have lower than expected aerobic capacity and physical performance, and their overall muscle strength is 60% below that of age-matched control subjects," concluding that "such patients tolerate well-tailored strengthening and endurance programs, with gains in physical performance levels in as brief a time as six weeks" [21]. Long-term exercise regimens in rheumatoid arthritis patients over many years have proved to be well tolerated with resultant improvement in functional and other outcome measures [22].

Because patients with arthritis have decreased endurance, these individuals should participate in some form of aerobic exercise to enhance their overall fitness. Studies have demonstrated the benefits of aerobic exercise for many conditions, including fibromyalgia pain [23], rheumatoid arthritis [24,25], lupus [26], and osteoarthritis [27]. Hampson and colleagues found that arthritic patients participating in exercise programs are more likely to effectively manage their osteoarthritic symptoms through low-impact exercise than with medications [28].

The properties of the aquatic environment make aquatic exercise and swimming (forms of low-impact exercise) good ways to manage arthritic symptoms. This contention has been substantiated in two studies of patient groups with non-acute rheumatoid and osteoarthritis participating in water exercise. In a Danish study, Danneskiold-Samsøe and coworkers found markedly increased isometric and isokinetic muscle strength of the quadriceps in rheumatoid subjects after only moderate training in the pool [29]. Other gains included an increase in aerobic capacity and freedom of movement and a higher degree of self-help in activities of daily living. Bunning and Materson found pool therapy to be effective for osteoarthritic patients, concluding that aquatic exercise should be the cornerstone of treatment for severe arthritis [27]. Patients who participated in the study exhibited significant improvements in aerobic capacity, ambulation distances, and physical activity levels. The use of group exercise also allowed increased socialization, counteracting the isolation that many arthritic patients feel. The overall benefits of aquatic exercise programs can include reduction of joint swelling; a decrease in joint stiffness and muscle soreness, which enhances the opportunities for active motion; improvement or maintenance of joint flexibility; increased muscle strength; improved coordination; increased endurance; and improved ability to perform daily tasks.

Aquatic therapy programs in a heated pool are effective for the arthritic for many reasons: Water's remarkable properties of heat transmission, buoyancy, resistance, and hydrostatic pressure provide a medium in which passive and voluntary exercise can be carried out with minimal stress and freedom, producing multiple therapeutic benefits. These biological effects are well described in earlier chapters.

Immersion and exercise in water of therapeutic temperatures (92–96°F) facilitates relaxation and the stretching and strengthening of muscles, ligaments, and tendons. Water has a very high capacity for specific heat, which means it absorbs or transfers heat very efficiently. Application of heat produces the following benefits in arthritic conditions:

- Increased collagen extensibility in tendons [30]
- Decreased joint stiffness [31]
- Pain relief [32]
- Pain threshold elevation [33]
- Muscle spasm relief [34]
- Increased circulation [35]
- Increased diuresis and cell metabolism [36]

Although warm water has been the traditional means of treating arthritic patients, and research has validated its utility, more recent surprising research has shown clinical results from cool-water immersion. Japanese researcher Nobunaga and coworkers [37] at Kyushu University studied the effects of cold-water bathing (13°C) on activity indices of morning stiffness and joint pain, grip strength, ease with activities of daily living, plasma norepinephrine levels, serum adrenocorticotropic hormone and cortisol levels, and a number of measures of immunosuppression. Significant gains in the activity indices were noted, along with significant elevations of norepinephrine. A mild immunosuppressive effect was noted in the cold-water population, with lowered immune complexes and lymphocyte subgroups. The control group, which had bathed in warm water (40°C) for comparable times, showed similar index reduction curves but lower performance levels throughout the treatment sessions. Only slight elevation of norepinephrine was noted in the warm-water control group and no immunosuppressive effect was found.

Water's buoyancy offsets body weight and supports painful and weakened structures. The density of water supports the immersed human body. When submerged to neck level, a person's apparent body weight is about one-tenth of his or her land weight, which enables the individual with weakness to move more comfortably. People with atrophied muscles are allowed complete freedom of movement due to their virtual weightlessness. When gradation of weight-bearing activities is desired, exercise can begin in deep water, where the lower extremities carry no weight and buoyancy unloads the compressive forces on the spine. For gradual increase in weight bearing, activities can be moved to progressively more shallow water. Patients recovering from lower-extremity joint replacement surgery, such as total hip replacement and total knee replacement, benefit tremendously from this approach. Passive ROM movements to prevent joint deformities and contractures are much easier to conduct in the aquatic environment. The use of buoyancy can be structured to assist, support, or resist motions of the extremities or trunk while ambient body weight is reduced. Water's viscosity acts as resistance to movement. As turbulence and speed of movement increase, so does resistance. The patient can use lightly resistive aquatic equipment to develop muscle strength and endurance.

Hydrostatic pressure assists in edema reduction. Edema, a major symptom of rheumatic conditions, can stretch intra-articular joint structures and produce pressure in the joint capsule. The pressure of periarticular edema is one of the factors that triggers pain with joint movement, which is a key factor in the initial loss of ROM and the development of joint stiffness.

The benefits available through whirlpool therapy are increased through the use of the larger therapeutic pool, which permits

- Simultaneous treatment of multiple joint problems
- Deeper immersion in the vertical position
- Heat transference through total body immersion
- A much broader range of therapeutic exercise
- Swimming for conditioning
- Ambulation training
- Use of popular spa techniques, such as the Bad Ragaz ring method (BRRM)
- Cost-effective group treatments versus more costly one-on-one therapy treatments

Given the current trends in population aging and the high age-related incidence of arthritis in our society, the construction of more therapeutic pools might be one of America's most worthwhile undertakings.

PROGRAMS

The aquatic environment presents a cost-effective and versatile option for occupational and physical therapists to expedite the goals of rehabilitation for a disease so pervasive as arthritis. Medically supervised water therapy interventions are available to the arthritic individual. The primary goals of treatment are the same for most of the rheumatic diseases:

- Mobilization of joints
- Strengthening of muscles
- Conditioning
- Re-education of function
- Patient education about activity pacing, joint protection, and disease management
- Instruction in self-directed exercise regimens

Aquatic therapy techniques are not simply adaptations of conventional land-based therapeutic exercise programs. The aquatic environment allows a different approach to achievement of therapeutic goals for a variety of arthritic conditions, using water's properties of buoyancy, heat absorption, pain reduction, and resistance to assist rehabilitative goals at each stage of the arthritic process. The approach is determined by whether the condition is acute, subacute, or chronic; inflammatory or noninflammatory; and unifocal or multifocal. Other considerations specific to the individual diagnosis also affect the management approach.

Acute Arthritis Management

Traditional medical management for acute episodes or flares consists of rest, immobilization, and medication for pain. Some evidence has surfaced in acute rheumatoid patients undergoing partial weight-bearing water exercise that regular exercise can decrease joint pain and inflammatory activity [38]. This effect may be due to endorphin release and in part to edema reduction. In the acute stages, therefore, gentle ROM exercise, strengthening, and endurance goals can be pursued in the therapeutic pool along with the passive benefits of pain relief, muscle relaxation, and decreased joint stresses. Uninvolved joints can also be exercised, and joints in a less acute phase may show therapeutic benefit.

In acute flares, some modifications of aquatic therapy technique are recommended. These include keeping the number of repetitions low (three to five repetitions), with therapist supervision or positioning to keep buoyancy or active patient motions from forcing the joints into extreme ROM. In the acute phase of treatment, it is important to educate the patient on joint protection principles in the use of equipment, handrails, and grab bars. Because movement is easier in water due to the lack of weight on joints and reduced pain, there can be a tendency to overdo; therefore, it is important to pace the activity and keep sessions short to avoid overfatiguing the patient. The patient should be counseled that if pain occurs after treatment and the pain persists for a period of hours or into the next day, exercise ranges and repetitions should be decreased. In the case of severe cervical joint involvement, use a Plastizote collar or a mask and snorkel in prone horizontal activities and swimming to prevent pain, cervical joint hypermobility, or even subluxation. When patients are febrile with a temperature elevation of more than 1°C, admission into the therapeutic pool is generally not advisable.

Subacute and Chronic Arthritis Management

Treatment programs for subacute and chronic cases can include one-on-one techniques with the therapist as well as more general exercises and activities designed to improve functional capacity. These include passive mobilization and relaxation; buoyancy-assisted, -supported, or -resisted exercise; and strength training, conditioning, and functional training for posture, balance, and mobility. Patients may be positioned in the seated, standing, horizontal supine, or prone flotation positions or suspended in deep water. Treatment may be carried out on an individual basis or in groups.

Mobilization of Joints

The goal of mobilization of joints and stretching muscles, ligaments, and tendons is common to many treatment protocols recommended for arthritic patients [39]. ROM exercises can help maintain joint movement, relieve stiffness, promote synovial fluid production and quality, and restore flexibility. The buoyancy and warmth of the water promote both general and specific relaxation of the muscle groups around painful joints [40]. Once the patient achieves this optimal state, exercise can progress from passive ROM movements performed by the therapist, to active assisted ROM exercise, to active patient exercise, and then to resistive exercise.

Passive Techniques

Mobilization of joints with contractures involves stretching fibrous tissue, but care must be taken not to overstretch periarticular structures, which may cause local recurrence of pain and inflammation [17]. It is essential that the therapist control joint mobilization techniques as well as limit range and activity in a specific joint. Receiving feedback from the patient about the effects of the last treatment is essential. After a session of joint mobilization, one can expect the joint to be a little sore for a few hours, but this should subside within 24 hours. Ron Harrison said, "In a joint that is both stiff and painful, the only way the therapist can be assured of achieving the desired effect is by isolating the movement with adequate fixation" [41]. This may mean positioning the patient on a pool chair, bench, or water plinth or working with a patient in a flotation setup with the therapist providing stabilization, as in the BRRM. Joint mobilization and joint oscillations can then be performed with accuracy.

Halliwick method techniques (e.g., rocking, swaying, snaking) may also be incorporated into passive treatment sessions to promote patient relaxation and elongation and traction to the spine and to decrease muscle guarding and splinting before exercise.

Active Assisted Exercise

In active assisted exercise, the individual moves the limb actively but may need some assistance in moving it through its full excursion. Treatment programs should begin with one-on-one techniques with the therapist, who can position the patient for best use of buoyancy and assist the limb through controlled available joint ROM. BRRM exercise using proximally controlled handholds is excellent for this purpose.

Active Exercise

In active exercise, the patient can move the body or body part through the water with control throughout the available joint ROM. General exercises and activities based on improving functional patterns of motion can be performed independently in specific positioning setups or in groups in the shallow water. Improving coordination of precise functional motions, with supervision and cueing as to proper use of body mechanics and joint protection principles is perhaps best done in the water. The therapist can readily observe spinal alignment and movement patterns in functional tasks, while the density and viscosity of the water slows down movements for observation and analysis. Many types of arthritis cause deformities that alter normal biomechanical alignment, and therefore postural deviations are quite common. The therapist is present to provide skilled corrections and modifications of active exercise. From poolside, careful attention to true body position is essential because the refractive properties of the water may create distortion that masks actual body posture. This is an argument for the therapist to stay in the pool until the patient is able to self-correct. Calisthenic exercises, water walking, deep-water exercises, and swimming instruction are modes of active exercise.

Resistive Exercise

Because water has buoyancy, movement is easier due to weight off-loading, but it becomes more difficult against the resistance presented by the viscosity of the water. This resistance varies, depending on such factors as the speed of movement, the surface area of the moving body part, the use of equipment, and the ambient turbulence of the water. The resistance noted with increasing speed of movement is not linear but complex and logarithmic. Viscous damping properties of water make the resistance drop almost instantaneously on cessation of effort. Water offers the arthritic the opportunity for protected, subtle, and gradable increases in resistive exercise to increase muscle strength and muscular endurance. When the body is submerged to

Table 5-1. Sample Progress Report: Upper-Body Aquatic Endurance Exercises

Date	Buoyancy Object	Number of Repetitions	Elapsed Time (min)	Movement Arc (degrees)
10/01/96	Small paddles	20 extensions	80	90–150
10/08/96	Large paddles	10 extensions	75	90–140
10/15/96	Quart jug	15 extensions	55	90–170

the neck, the effect of gravity on joints with impaired integrity is negligible. Muscles can be strengthened through isometric exercises by holding a stable position against the resistance of the water, against therapist-created turbulence, against a float, or by maintaining a static position while being pushed through the water, as in certain patterns of the BRRM. By moving the body or limb through water, the patient can perform isokinetic resistive exercise to strengthen muscles. Because water is a three-dimensional medium, active exercise in any direction is resistive. A wide variety of aquatic exercise equipment is available to grade and progress the activity. Light weight training of three to 10 repetitions in specific muscle groups is indicated to minimize the debilitating effects of many arthritic conditions and for the development and maintenance of lean muscle mass. Graded isokinetic water activities provide a protective medium to accomplish this aim. It is important to slow the speed of movement through the ROM whenever equipment is added to prevent injury.

BRRM and conventional water exercises performed under a therapist's supervision are also effective in the treatment of patient weakness [1]. Conventional water exercise uses flotation rings, which act as added resistance when the patient performs a motion against the force of buoyancy. This method may generate considerable resistance to the muscles, depending on the buoyant object. The exercise effort may be graded by using progressively buoyant objects, increasing the number of repetitions, speeding up the movement, and going through larger arcs of movement. Table 5-1 is an example of a grid that might be used to quantify progress.

It is important to quantify exercise movement in arthritis because patients need protection against overload, which requires knowledge of past loads successfully managed. In this way strength is developed while joint tolerances are monitored. The faster the motion away from buoyancy or the more air in the flotation rings, the greater the resistance to movement (Figure 5-2). In BRRM exercises, the therapist acts as a fixator around which the patient works isometrically, supported by floats in supine, prone, or side-lying positions, while moving in straight or diagonal closed chains of movement (Figures 5-3 and 5-4). Thus, the arms, trunk, and legs can be strengthened using a system of resistance progression readily graded by the aquatic therapist trained in this method. A word of precaution: When working with patients who have abnormal joint physiology, the therapist must keep the momentum of initiated movements from proceeding too far by stepping forward into the direction of the joint movement when the movement approaches end ranges (Figure 5-5).

Aerobic Conditioning

Paramount to the prevention and slowing of the progression of many arthritic diseases is the control of joint loading [2]. Water provides a safe, versatile, and protective medium for the deconditioned individual to initiate or enhance his or her cardiovascular capacity. A wide variety of aerobic exercise modes can be

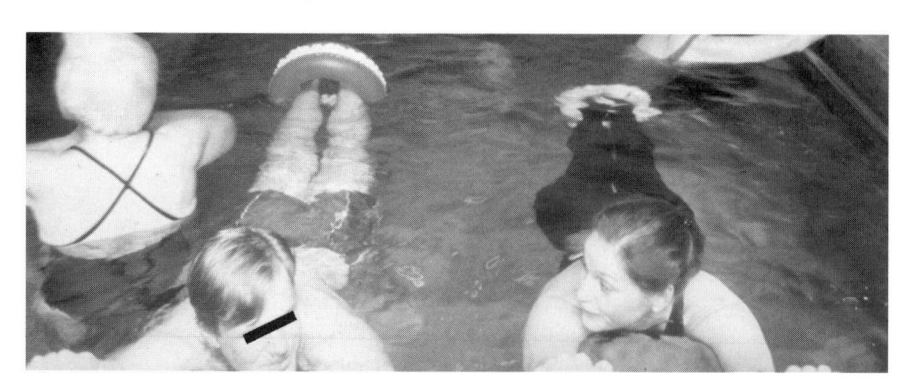

Figure 5-2. Resistive water exercise against flotation in a water ring. (Courtesy of Aquatic Rehabilitation Consultants, Smithfield, VA.)

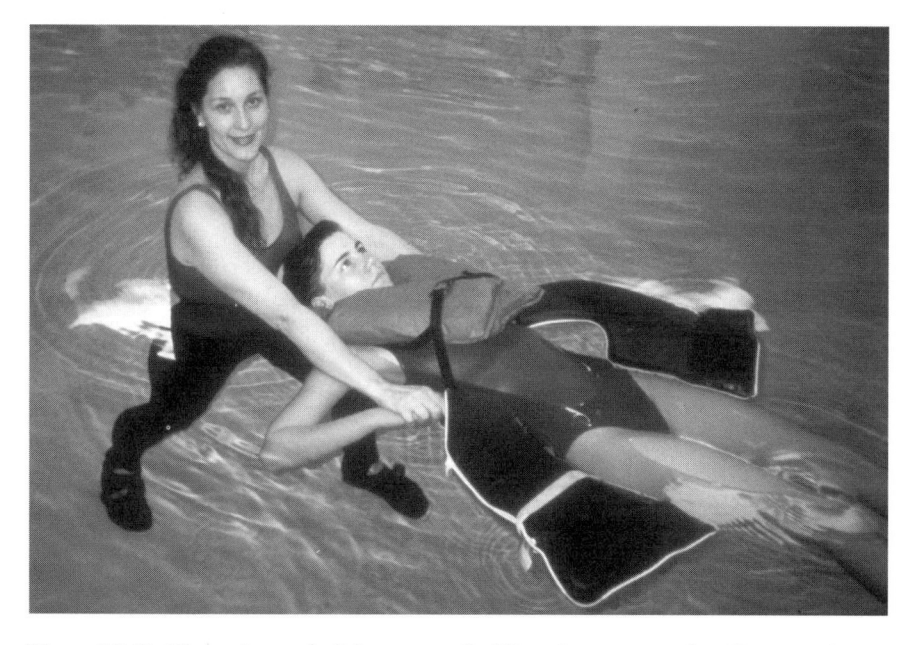

Figure 5-3. Bad Ragaz ring method. Arm pattern for bilateral upper extremity. (Courtesy of Aquatic Rehabilitation Consultants, Smithfield, VA.)

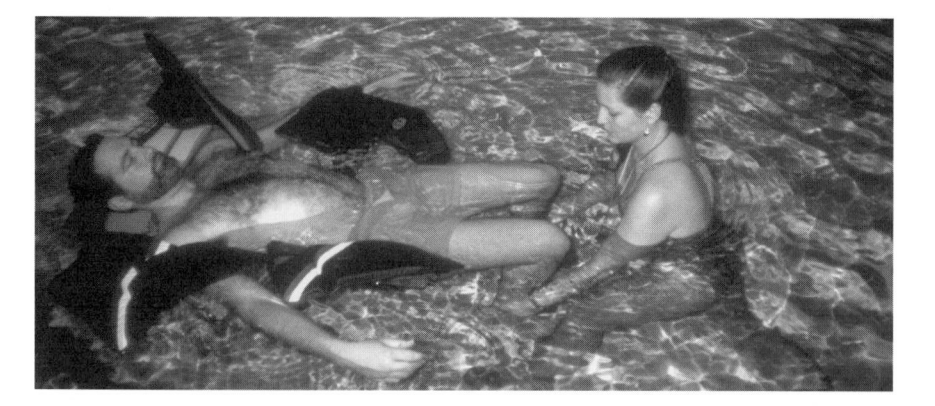

Figure 5-4. Bad Ragaz ring method. Leg pattern for bilateral knee flexion. (Courtesy of Aquatic Rehabilitation Consultants, Smithfield, VA.)

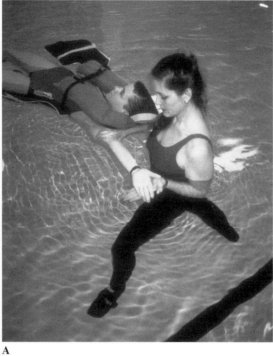

A

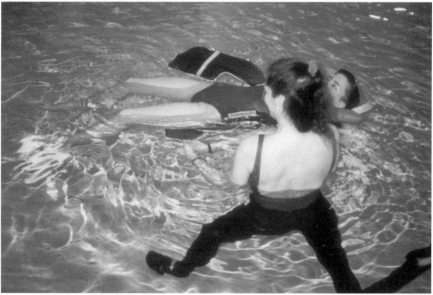

B

Figure 5-5. Therapist breaking resistance in Bad Ragaz arm pattern by stepping in the direction of the patient's motion. A. Starting motion. B. Ending motion. (Courtesy of Aquatic Rehabilitation Consultants, Smithfield, VA.)

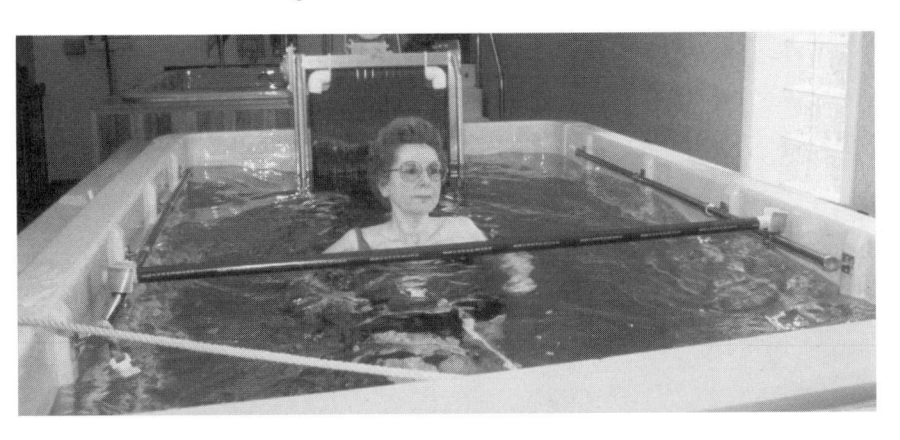

Figure 5-6. Rheumatoid arthritic patient exercising in a water tank. (Courtesy of Aqua ARK, Inc., Doylestown, PA.)

conducted in water of varying depths. Deep-water exercise, in which the patient can be suspended with a flotation belt, saddle, or vest in the vertical position at the water's surface, permits a wide range of non-weight-bearing underwater exercise that can be aerobically formatted (Figure 5-6). Some examples are water running, scissor kicks, cross-country skiing movements, abduction-adduction kicks with and without lower-extremity water resistance equipment such as fins and boots with simultaneous upper-extremity motions of figure-eights, finning, and sculling. Aerobic conditioning of very high intensity can be accomplished even while protecting injured joints.

Shallow water also offers a range of aerobic workout opportunities, such as water walking (Figure 5-7), water aerobics in which calisthenics are performed in simple straight planes of motion incorporating good body mechanics, and exercising with lightly resistive aquatic equipment. Swimming with adaptations made for adherence to proper postural alignment and joint protection techniques is yet another aquatic aerobic option for the rheumatic patient. For specific problems, the therapist can design aquatic aerobic circuits using functional tolerances and motions, such as squatting to standing, sitting to standing, trunk flexion to extension, and ambulation (Figure 5-8).

Re-Education of Function

Improvement and maintenance of joint flexibility, muscle strength, and cardiovascular conditioning improve physical capacity, which translates into improved function. Measurable functional outcome activities, such as supine rolling, coming from supine to sitting, sitting balance, upper-extremity movement in sitting, moving from sitting to standing, standing balance, ambulation for flat and uneven terrain, and stair climbing, can be done effectively with skilled therapeutic aquatic therapy intervention. First, the patient performs the activity in the water and then progresses to land under gravity load. Restoration of the muscles' normal pattern of movement with freedom from pain is the functional outcome measure from which to judge the effectiveness of treatment interventions.

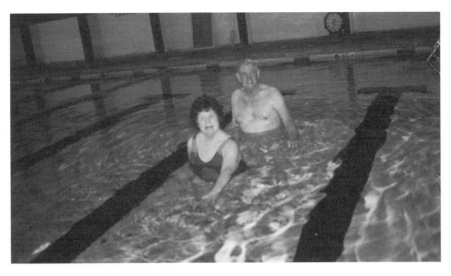

Figure 5-7. Osteoarthritic patients water walking. (Courtesy of Aquatic Rehabilitation Consultants, Smithfield, VA.)

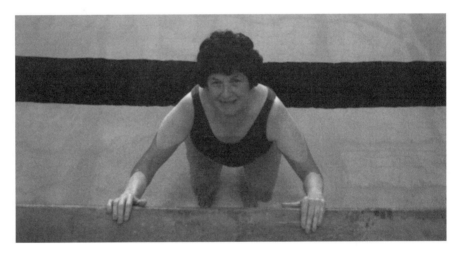

Figure 5-8. Total knee replacement patient performing squats in the pool. (Courtesy of Aquatic Rehabilitation Consultants, Smithfield, VA.)

PATIENT EDUCATION

Joint Protection, Pacing, and Management

Exercise groups and aquatic circuits lend themselves well to educationally formatted group treatments, which are cost effective, offer psychological and peer support, and emphasize important patient educational goals. Pacing, joint protection skills, proper body mechanics, pain management, and self-empowering knowledge of exercise theory can be taught effectively in groups with the goal of long-term maintenance and independent exercise program adherence [42]. Such groups may facilitate exercise adherence while decreasing health care system use and its associated costs.

Community Transitioning

Once discharged from skilled water therapy and rehabilitation programs, patients with arthritis should follow some type of functional maintenance program. Recognizing the importance of water exercise for those who suffer from arthritis, the Arthritis Foundation in cooperation with the YMCA has developed a nationwide Arthritis Aquatics Program. This carefully structured recreational program has incorporated the basic tenets of arthritic precautions so that a safe, effective, low-cost, and medically sound water exercise program is available to those with arthritis. Certification in the content base is available for interested therapists, and training materials are available through the foundation (1330 W. Peachtree Street, Atlanta, GA 30309). Information regarding the nearest Arthritis Aquatics Program may be located through the arthritis information line at 800-283-7800. The original program was developed in 1983 and was revised in 1990 and 1996. It uses 68 ROM and strengthening exercises and an optional endurance-building component; several are shown in the chapter appendix. Swimming skills are unnecessary. The certification process is sufficient so that a medical practitioner may generally feel comfortable referring a patient to the program, and the author's experience has been that patient adherence has been high, therapeutic value significant, and cost to the patient low. The Arthritis Foundation has developed two other programs, PACE (People with Arthritis Can Exercise), a community-based group program, and Joint Efforts, a gentle exercise program for sedentary older adults.

The PACE program consists of calisthenic exercises in straight planes of motion that promote total body flexibility and gentle aerobic exercises that increase cardiovascular capacity. Water walking, deep-water exercise, and swimming are aerobic modes from which individuals can select (Figures 5-9 and 5-10).

CONCLUSION

The physical properties of water create an ideal environment for the rehabilitation of the arthritic patient, as has been known and practiced since the beginning of recorded medical therapeutics. Watching the relief on a patient's face as he or she slips into warm water allows no other conclusion. These physical properties of water address nearly all the causes of arthritic symptoms and allow the patient an opportunity to reduce pain, decrease joint swelling, increase joint movement and strength, and preserve and build functional capacity while in a comfortable relaxing medium. The therapeutic options range from simple warm water immersion, to passive and active underwater exercise techniques, to skilled hydrotherapeutic interventions by an aquatic therapist in individual and group treatments. These therapies can progress into recreational usage of water for exercise maintenance. The therapeutic margin of safety is exceedingly high, permitting self-directed exercise programs and low-cost disease management. The aquatic options beneficial to management of the arthritic individual are nearly endless, depending only on the imagination and creativity of the individual with arthritis and his or her therapist or physician.

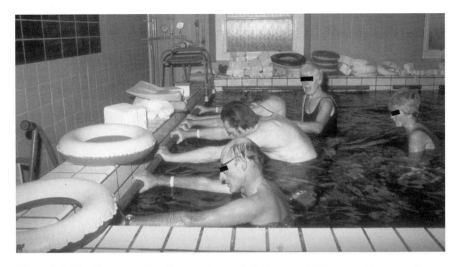

Figure 5-9. Shoulder range of motion exercises: ankylosing spondylitis group. (Courtesy of Aquatic Rehabilitation Consultants, Smithfield, VA.)

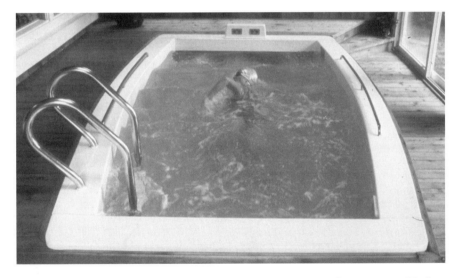

Figure 5-10. Swimming against a gradable resistant current. (Courtesy of Swimex, Inc., Warrington, RI.)

REFERENCES

1. Harrison RA. Hydrotherapy in Rheumatic Conditions. In SA Hyde (ed), Physiotherapy in Rheumatology. Oxford: Blackwell, 1980.
2. Reed KL. Quick Reference to Occupational Therapy. Rockville, MD: Aspen, 1991.
3. Freeman MAR. Operative Surgery in Rheumatic Diseases. In M Mason, HLF Curry (eds), Clinical Rheumatology. Philadelphia: Lippincott, 1970.
4. Mosby's Medical, Nursing, and Allied Health Dictionary (4th ed). Philadelphia: Mosby–Year Book, 1994.
5. Scott DL. Rest or exercise in inflammatory arthritis. Br J Hosp Med 1992;48:445.
6. Robinson D. Osteoarthritis. In ME Rubenstein, DD Federman (eds), Scientific American Medicine. New York: Scientific American, 1994;1.
7. Verbrugge LM, Patrick DL. Seven chronic conditions and their impact on U.S. adults' activity levels and use of medical services. Am J Public Health 1995;85:173.
8. Marmer L. Preparing for the arthritis epidemic. Occup Ther Adv 1995;11:12, 13, 54.
9. Centers for Disease Control. Morbidity & Mortality World Report. Atlanta, GA: Centers for Disease Control, June 24, 1994.
10. Guccione AA. Arthritis and the process of disablement. Phys Ther 1994;74:408.
11. Caspers J, Ostle E. Osteoarthritis and Rheumatoid Arthritis. In M Helm (ed), Occupational Therapy with the Elderly. New York: Churchill Livingstone, 1987;31.
12. Instill J. Reconstructive Surgery and Rehabilitation of the Knee. In WM Kelly, ED Harris, S Ruddy, CB Sledge (eds), Arthritis and Related Disorders. Philadelphia: Saunders, 1981.
13. deAndre JR, Grant C, Dixon AS. Joint distension and reflex muscle inhibition in the knee. J Bone Joint Surg Am 1965;47:313.
14. Herbison GJ, Ditunno J, Jaweed M. Muscle atrophy in rheumatoid arthritis. J Rheumatol 1987;14(Suppl 15):78.
15. Danneskiold-Samsøe B, Grimby G. The relationship between leg muscle strength and physical capacity in patients with rheumatoid arthritis with reference to the influence of corticosteroids. Clin Rheumatol 1986;5:468.
16. Hicks JE. Exercise in patients with inflammatory arthritis and connective tissue disease. Rheum Dis Clin North Am 1990;16:845.
17. Swezey RL. Rehabilitation Aspects in Arthritis. In DJ McCarty (ed), Arthritis and Related Disorders (9th ed). Philadelphia: Lea & Febiger, 1979;349.
18. Melvin JL. Rheumatic Disease in the Adult and Child: Occupational Therapy and Rehabilitation (3rd ed). Philadelphia: Davis, 1989.
19. Gerber LH. Principles and Their Application in Rehabilitation of Patients with Rheumatic Diseases. In WM Kelly, ED Harris, S Ruddy, CB Sledge (eds), Arthritis and Related Disorders. Philadelphia: Saunders, 1981.
20. Namey TC (ed). Exercise and arthritis. Rheum Dis Clin North Am 1990;16:1, 832, 1023.
21. Beals C. A case for aerobic conditioning exercise in rheumatoid arthritis [abstract]. Clin Res 1981;29:780A.
22. Nordemar R. Physical training in rheumatoid arthritis: a controlled long-term study. II. Functional capacity and general attitudes. Scand J Rheumatol 1981;10:25.
23. McCain G. Non-medical treatment in primary myalgia. Rheum Dis Clin North Am 1989;15:73.
24. Ekdahl C, Anderson SI, Mortotz V, et al. Dynamic versus static training in patients with rheumatoid arthritis. Scand J Rheumatol 1990;19:17.
25. Perlman SG, Connell K, Alberti J, et al. Synergistic effects of exercise and problem solving education for rheumatoid arthritis patients. Arthritis Rheum 1987;30(Suppl):13.
26. Robb-Nicholson C, Daltroy E, Eaton H, et al. Effects of aerobic conditioning in lupus fatigue: a pilot study. Br J Rheumatol 1989;28:500.
27. Bunning RD, Materson RS. A rational program of exercise for patients with osteoarthritis. Semin Arthritis Rheum 1991;21(Suppl):33.
28. Hampson SE, Glosgow RE, Zeiss AM, et al. A self management of osteoarthritis. Arthritis Care Res 1993;6:17.

29. Danneskiold-Samsøe B, Lyngberg K, Risum T, Telling M. The effects of water exercise therapy given to patients with rheumatoid arthritis. Scand J Rehabil Med 1987;19:31.
30. Gersten JW. Effects of ultrasound on tendon extensibility. Am J Phys Med 1995;34:362.
31. Bucklund L, Tiselius P. Objective measurement of joint stiffness in rheumatoid arthritis. Acta Rheumatoid Scand 1967;13:275.
32. Harris E Jr, McCroskery PA. The influence of temperature and fibril stability on degradation of cartilage collagen by rheumatoid synovial collagenase. N Engl J Med 1974;290:1.
33. Benson TB, Copp EP. The effects of therapeutic forms of heat and ice on the pain threshold of the normal shoulder. Rheumatol Rehabil 1974;13:101.
34. Don Figny R, Sheldon K. Simultaneous use of heat and cold in the treatment of muscle spasm. Arch Phys Med Rehabil 1962;43:235.
35. Harris PR. Iontophoresis: clinical research in musculoskeletal inflammatory conditions. J Orthop Sports Phys Ther 1982;4:109.
36. Epstein M. Renal effects of head out immersion in humans: a 15-year update. Physiol Rev 1992;72:563.
37. Nobunaga M, Tatsukawa K, Ishii H, Yoshida F. Balneotherapy for Patients with Rheumatoid Arthritis, Especially the Effect of Cold Spring Water Bathing. In Y Agishi, Y Ohtsuka (eds), New Frontiers in Health Resort Medicine. Noboribetsu, Japan: Hokkaido University School of Medicine Press, 1996;109.
38. Scott DL. Rest or exercise in inflammatory arthritis. Br J Hosp Med 1992;48:445.
39. Melvin JL. Rheumatic Disease: Occupational Therapy and Rehabilitation. Philadelphia: Davis, 1980.
40. Pennington FC. Water exercise can provide relief for people with arthritis. Dealer News 1990;19.
41. Harrison RA. Hydrotherapy in arthritis. Practitioner 1972;208:132.
42. Becker BE. Motivating adherence in the rehabilitation setting. J Back Musculoskel Med 1991;1:37.

Appendix 5.1
Arthritis Foundation YMCA Aquatics Program Class Planner Worksheet 1

SAMPLE PROGRAM

Exercise Category	Exercise Number	Suggested Name	Comments
Walking, 5-min warm-up	1	Forward	
	2	Backward	
	5	Sidestepping	
Neck exercise	10	Neck rotation	
	11	Neck tilts	
Shoulder exercise	17	Shoulder circles	
	16	Shoulder shrugs	
	18	Flexion/extension	
	22	Abduction/adduction	
	27	Internal/external rotation	
	35	Rope pull	
Trunk stretching exercise	12	Side bends	
Elbow exercise	37	Flexion/extension	
Hip and knee exercise	51	Quadriceps stretch	
	53	Hip and knee	
	55	Flex/extension squats	
	62	Calf stretch	
	59	Leg circles	

Source: Adapted with permission from YMCA Aquatics Instructors Manual. AFYAP Program Institute, Arthritis Foundation, Alpharetta, GA.

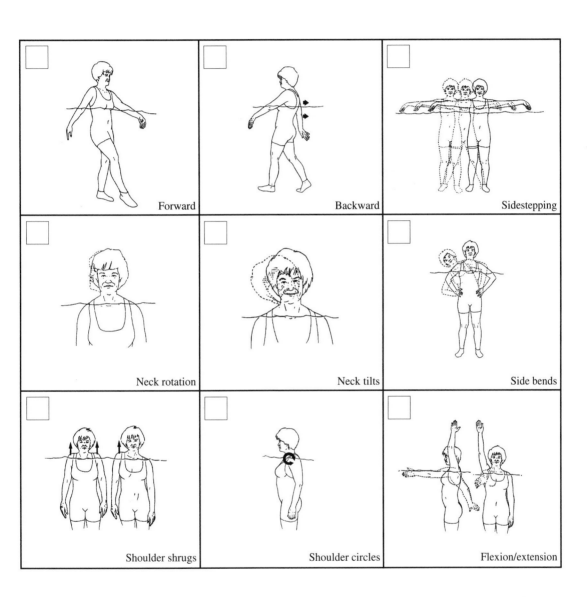

Forward

Backward

Sidestepping

Neck rotation

Neck tilts

Side bends

Shoulder shrugs

Shoulder circles

Flexion/extension

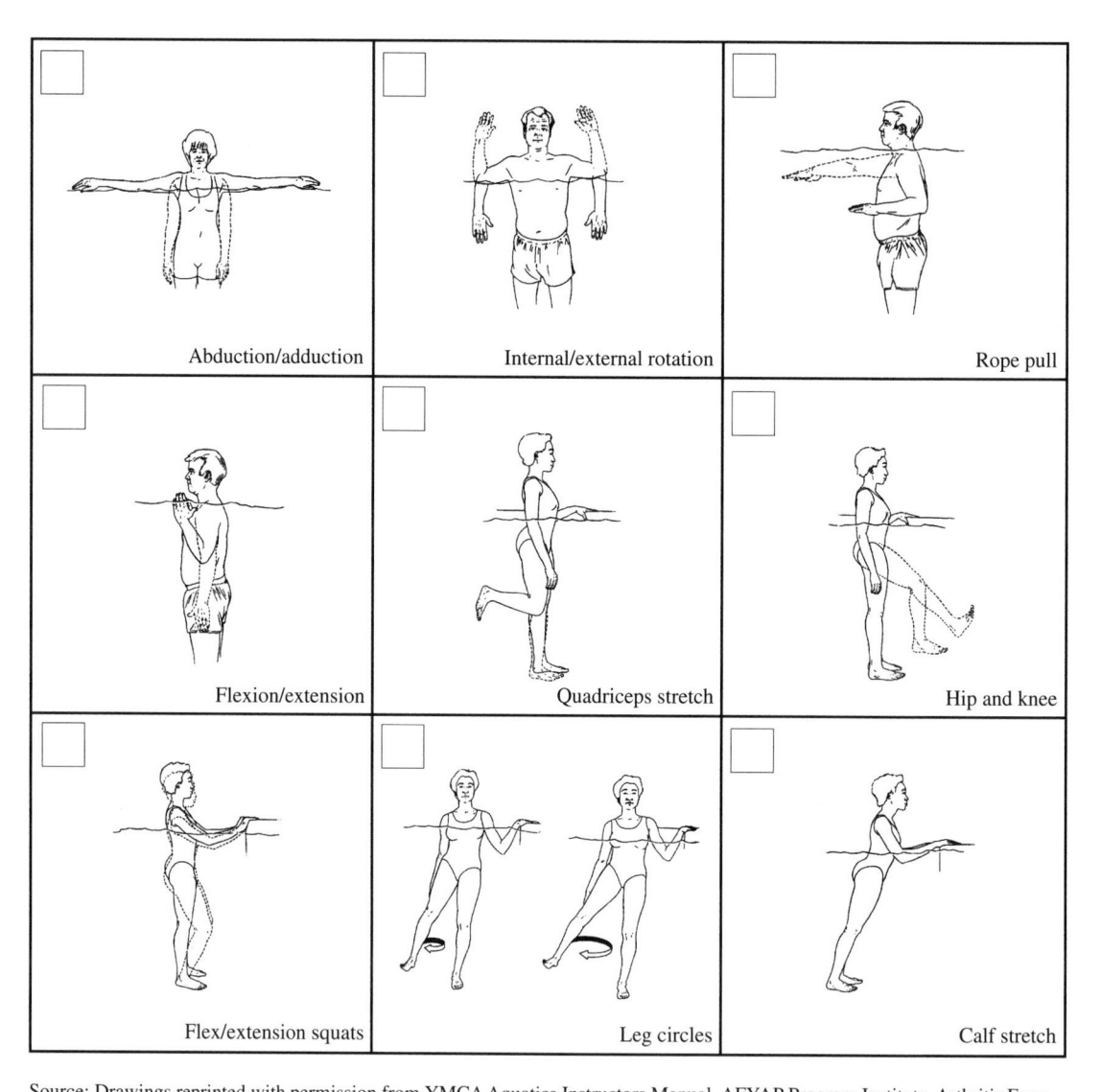

Abduction/adduction	Internal/external rotation	Rope pull
Flexion/extension	Quadriceps stretch	Hip and knee
Flex/extension squats	Leg circles	Calf stretch

Source: Drawings reprinted with permission from YMCA Aquatics Instructors Manual. AFYAP Program Institute. Arthritis Foundation, Alpharetta, GA.

6

Techniques of Aqua Running

Robert P. Wilder and David K. Brennan

Aqua running is an effective form of cardiovascular conditioning. Sufficient cardiovascular response has been demonstrated to result in a training effect. Understanding the bioengineering principles of the aquatic environment, proper technique, physiologic response, and methods of exercise prescription helps practitioners to incorporate aqua running into rehabilitation and training programs.

Deep-water exercise is being used in the treatment and conditioning programs for a number of rehabilitation populations. This is especially true in the field of sports medicine, where aqua running is used as an effective form of cardiovascular conditioning for injured athletes as well as for others who desire a low-impact aerobic workout. Aqua running, or deep-water running, consists of simulated running in the deep end of a pool aided by a flotation device (vest or belt) that maintains the head above water. The participant may be held in one location by a tether cord, essentially running in place, or may actually run through the water across the width of the pool. The tether serves to increase resistance, to assist in maintaining a near vertical posture, and to facilitate monitoring of exercise by a physician, therapist, or coach. No contact is made with the bottom of the pool, thus eliminating impact. The elimination of weight load on joints makes this an ideal method for rehabilitating or conditioning injured athletes, particularly those with foot, ankle, or knee injuries for whom running on land is contraindicated.

PRINCIPLES OF HYDROTHERAPY

Several properties of water make it an ideal environment for exercise [1].

Buoyancy

Buoyancy supports a body submerged in water, counteracting the downward pull of gravity. The submerged body seems to lose weight equal to the weight of the water displaced, resulting in less stress and pressure on bone, muscle, and connective tissue.

Drag Force

The viscosity and drag force of water provide a resistance proportional to the effort exerted, much like running into a stiff wind. This adds to the cardiovascular challenge of aquatic exercise without creating impact stress on joints and soft tissue.

Hydrostatic Pressure

Hydrostatic pressure (i.e., pressure exerted by water on a submerged body) is proportional to depth and is equal in all directions. It is thought to aid cardiovascular function by promoting venous return.

Specific Heat

Specific heat is the amount of heat needed to raise the temperature of a substance by 1°C. The specific heat of water is several times that of air; therefore, the rate of heat loss in water is much greater than the rate of heat loss to air at the same temperature. This is an especially important consideration in warmer climates, where heat illness is a significant source of morbidity. It is also helpful in training injured athletes who are deconditioned and not acclimated to exercise in warm environments.

Temperature

The aquatic environment allows regulation of the temperature during exercise. An ideal range appears to be 82–86°F (28–30°C), in which little heat is stored and performance is not impaired. In our experience, competitive athletes typically prefer a slightly cooler environment.

BIOMECHANICS OF AQUA RUNNING

The form of running in water is patterned as closely as possible after that used on land (Figure 6-1). For the runner (or any athlete whose sport requires running), aqua running is therefore a biomechanically specific means of conditioning during a rehabilitation program or when supplementing regular training. This has special importance because the effects of training include not only improvement in cardiac and pulmonary performance but also improvement in muscle groups that undergo enzyme, capillary-density, and other adaptations to exercise. Compared to land-based running, the elimination of weight bearing and the addition of resistance in aqua running change the relative contribution of each muscle group. Every effort is made, therefore, to reproduce the running form used on land and to ensure the use of the same muscle groups.

The following guidelines help patients to maintain proper form during aqua running [2]:

- The water line should be at shoulder level. The mouth should be comfortably out of the water without cervical spine extension. The head should be looking straight ahead, with the neck unflexed.

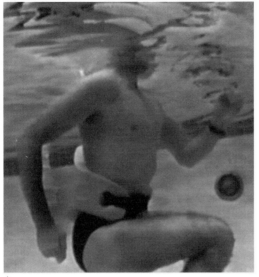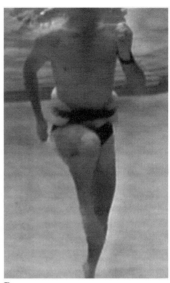

A   B

Figure 6-1. The form of running in water closely mimics the form used on land. Notice that the arm carriage is identical to that used with land-based running. A. Lateral view. B. Frontal view.

- The body should assume a position slightly forward of the vertical, with the spine maintained in a neutral position.
- Arm motion is identical to that used on land, with primary motion at the shoulder. Hands are held lightly clenched.
- Hip flexion should reach 60–80 degrees. As the hip is being flexed, the leg is extended at the knee (from the flexed position). When end-range hip flexion is reached, the lower leg should be perpendicular to the horizontal. The hip and knee are then extended together, the knee reaching full extension when the hip is in neutral position (i.e., 0 degrees flexion). As the hip is extended, the leg is flexed at the knee. These movements are repeated, and throughout the cycle, the ankle undergoes dorsiflexion and plantar flexion. The ankle is in a position of dorsiflexion when the hip is in neutral position and the leg extended at the knee. Plantar flexion is assumed as the hip is extended and the leg flexed. Dorsiflexion is reassumed as the hip is flexed and the leg extended. Underwater viewing demonstrates that inversion and eversion accompany dorsiflexion and plantar flexion, similar to land-based running.

EXERCISE RESPONSE TO AQUA RUNNING

The metabolic responses to aqua running and land-based running differ significantly [3]. Nonetheless, aqua running elicits sufficient cardiovascular response to result in a training effect, thus supporting anecdotal evidence of its usefulness in the rehabilitation of the athlete. The American College of Sports Medicine Guidelines for Exercise Prescription state that to obtain a training effect, exercise should be performed three to five times per week at an intensity level between 40% and 85% of maximum oxygen uptake ($\dot{V}O_{2max}$), or 55–90% of maximum heart rate. This level should

Table 6-1. Maximal Physiologic Responses (Mean [Standard Deviation]) to Deep-Water Running (DWR)

Physiologic Measure	Butts et al., 1991	Butts et al., 1991 (females)	Butts et al., 1991 (males)	Svegenhag and Seger, 1992	Town and Bradley, 1991	Navia, 1986
$\dot{V}O_{2max}$ TM (liters/min)	3.0 (0.3)	3.321 (0.317)	4.550 (0.368)	4.60 (0.14)	—	—
$\dot{V}O_{2max}$ DWR (liters/min)	2.6 (0.5)	2.786 (0.367)	4.086 (0.405)	4.03 (0.13)	—	—
$\dot{V}O_{2max}$ TM (ml/kg/min)	54.7 (7.0)	55.7 (4.8)	64.5 (2.8)	—	—	58
$\dot{V}O_{2max}$ DWR (ml/kg/min)	46.8 (9.1)	46.8 (5.9)	58.4 (3.9)	—	—	48
$\dot{V}O_{2max}$ DWR/TM (%)	86	84	89	87.8 (2.4)	73.50	83
HR max TM (bpm)	197.9 (9.4)	188.7 (9.3)	193.3 (5.8)	188 (2)	—	197
HR max DWR (bpm)	180.3 (6.0)	179.5 (7.5)	183.4 (5.9)	172 (3)	—	175
HR DWR/TM (%)	91	95	95	91	90	89
RER TM	1.05 (0.03)	1.13 (0.03)	1.15 (0.04)	1.2 (0.03)	—	—
RER DWR	1.01 (0.08)	1.09 (0.04)	1.11 (0.03)	1.1 (0.04)	—	0.95
RPE TM	19.1 (0.3)	—	—	—	—	19.2
RPE DWR	19.3 (0.6)	—	—	—	—	19.1
Lactate TM (mmol/liter)	—	—	—	10.0 (0.16)	—	—
Lactate DWR (mmol/liter)	—	—	—	12.4 (1.3)	—	—
Lactate DWR/TM (%)	—	—	—	124	81	—
O₂ pulse max TM (ml O₂/beat)	—	—	—	24.5	—	—
O₂ pulse max DWR (ml O₂/beat)	—	—	—	23.4	—	—
O₂ pulse max DWR/TM	—	—	—	0.096	—	—
Ventilation TM (liters/min)	—	111.6 (7.0)	150.0 (11.6)	—	—	—
Ventilation DWR (liters/min)	—	97.7 (10.9)	140.8 (17.8)	—	—	—

HR = heart rate; RER = respiratory exchange ratio; RPE = rating of perceived exertion; TM = treadmill.
Source: Reprinted with permission from RP Wilder, DK Brennan. Physiologic responses to deep water running in athletes. Sports Med 1993;16:374.

be maintained for 15–60 minutes [4]. Studies have demonstrated that aqua running elicits responses well within these suggested ranges.

Maximal Physiologic Responses

Several studies have compared the maximal physiologic responses to aqua running and land-based running (Table 6-1) [5–8]. Important measures of response to exercise of maximal intensity include $\dot{V}O_{2max}$ and maximal heart rate. $\dot{V}O_{2max}$ values during supported deep-water running (with a flotation device) are 83–89% of values obtained during land-based running. Heart rates during deep-water running range from 89% to 95% of values obtained during land-based running.

Butts et al. [5] reported results obtained during maximal graded exercise tests (GXTs) of deep-water running in 12 female high school cross-country runners. The average $\dot{V}O_{2max}$ during deep-water running was 86% of the average $\dot{V}O_{2max}$ obtained during a treadmill GXT. Peak heart rates averaged 91% of values obtained on the treadmill. No significant difference was noted in maximal perceived exertion. In a similar study, Butts et al. [6] examined maximal responses in 24 trained men and women. The average $\dot{V}O_{2max}$ values measured during a GXT of deep-water running were 84% of those obtained during treadmill running for women and 89% for men.

Peak heart rates during deep-water running averaged 95% of values obtained on land. Ventilation volumes also were found to be significantly lower during deep-water running. Men had significantly greater ventilation volume and $\dot{V}O_{2max}$ than women (as has been shown with land-based exercise); however, no significant difference between the sexes was noted for respiratory exchange ratio (RER) or peak heart rate.

During maximal-level deep-water running in 10 trained runners, Svedenhag and Seger [7] recorded $\dot{V}O_{2max}$ values averaging 88% and peak heart rates averaging 91% of values obtained during treadmill running. Blood lactate levels tended to be higher after maximal deep-water running (12.4 mmol/liter vs. 10.0 mmol/liter). Maximal oxygen pulse was slightly lower during deep-water running (23.4 ml oxygen per beat vs. 24.5 ml oxygen per beat). During a symptom-limited deep-water running GXT, Navia demonstrated $\dot{V}O_{2max}$ averaging 83% and peak heart rates averaging 89% of values attained during maximal treadmill running. The RER reported during deep-water running, however, averaged only 0.95, which is insufficient to qualify as a true maximal test (AM Navia, unpublished observation, 1986).

During unsupported deep-water running (without a flotation device), Town and Bradley [8] reported $\dot{V}O_{2max}$ averaging 73.5% and peak heart rates averaging 90% of those values obtained on land. Blood lactate levels after maximal deep-water running were lower than those levels after maximal treadmill running, but the water test lasted only 4 minutes (two 1-minute submaximal stages and a 2-minute stage at maximal intensity); treadmill stages lasted 3 minutes each. In our experience, 1-minute stages are insufficient to effect a complete response to a particular exercise intensity during deep-water running.

Submaximal Physiologic Responses

Important relationships between rate of perceived exertion (RPE), heart rate, and oxygen uptake ($\dot{V}O_2$) have also been noted during deep-water running at submaximal intensities. For a given level of perceived exertion, heart rates and $\dot{V}O_2$ levels tend to be lower during deep-water running than during treadmill running. In GXTs, Svedenhag and Seger [7] noted higher central and peripheral RPEs during deep-water running at any given $\dot{V}O_2$ or heart rate compared to treadmill running at the same intensity. Navia reported a similar relationship between RPE and physiologic responses during graded exercise. Higher RPE values were expressed during deep-water running at any given heart rate than during treadmill running. A similar relationship was noted for RPE and $\dot{V}O_2$. These differences should be noted if RPE is used as the sole measure of exercise intensity.

During submaximal deep-water running for 45 minutes, Bishop et al. [9] recorded lower mean $\dot{V}O_2$ rates and ventilation values than those recorded during a 45-minute treadmill run at a comparable perceived exertion ($\dot{V}O_2$ was 29.8 cc/kg/min vs. 40.6 cc/kg/min; ventilation was 58.1 liters/min vs. 79.1 liters/min). Heart rates were also lower during deep-water running (122 vs. 157 bpm); however, this was not deemed statistically significant with the small sample involved ($n = 7$). Two participants, who were described as the most accomplished and enthusiastic deep-water runners, achieved similar responses during deep-water running and treadmill running, suggesting that motivation or familiarity may play a role in attaining levels of physiologic response.

Ritchie and Hopkins [10] noted that perceived exertion and pain during a 30-minute deep-water run at a "hard" pace were comparable to those ratings obtained during "hard" treadmill running. These ratings were significantly greater than perceived exertion during treadmill running or road running at a "normal" training pace.

Examining the relationship between heart rate and $\dot{V}O_2$ during submaximal graded exercise, Svedenhag and Seger [7] reported lower heart rates during deep-water running than treadmill running at any given level of $\dot{V}O_2$. Oxygen pulse also was higher during submaximal exercise in water. A similar relationship between heart rate and $\dot{V}O_2$ was noted by Navia (unpublished observation, 1986) at higher work loads. These results suggest that an aerobic training effect may occur at lower heart rates during deep-water running than during treadmill running.

Yamaji et al. [11] noted significant interindividual variability in heart rate responses as a function of $\dot{V}O_2$ during unsupported deep-water running. Although group data revealed a similar heart rate–$\dot{V}O_2$ relationship for both deep-water running and treadmill running, two of the more skilled participants did have lower heart rate values during deep-water running than during treadmill running at a comparative $\dot{V}O_2$. Ritchie and Hopkins [10] obtained heart rate values during a 30-minute session of hard deep-water running that were lower than those during hard treadmill running (159 bpm vs. 176 bpm). $\dot{V}O_2$ values, however, were similar (49 ml/kg/min vs. 53 ml/kg/min). The heart rate values obtained during hard deep-water running were similar to those obtained during treadmill running at a normal training pace; however, corresponding $\dot{V}O_2$ was greater during hard deep-water running. This study also supports the contention that deep-water running may result in greater overall aerobic response if heart rate is used as the measure of exercise intensity.

Long-Term Training Effects

Four studies have reported the long-term effects of a deep-water exercise program. Michaud et al. [12] reported that 10 subjects who underwent an 8-week training program of aqua running showed improvements in $\dot{V}O_{2max}$ during both water-based and land-based graded exercise testing (19.6% and 10.7%, respectively), thus demonstrating a training effect as well as a crossover effect to land-based exercise. Eyestone et al. [13] demonstrated that deep-water running was comparable to land-based running and cycling for preserving levels of fitness during a 6-week training period at maintenance duration (20–30 minutes) and frequency (three to five times per week). Although a small decrease in $\dot{V}O_{2max}$ was noted for each group, this was much less than the 16–17% loss previously reported during a 6-week rest period.

Wilber et al. [14] demonstrated no significant differences in treadmill $\dot{V}O_{2max}$, ventilatory threshold, running economy, and blood lactate at $\dot{V}O_{2max}$ after 6 weeks of training in two groups, one training on land, the other training exclusively in water. Additionally, glucose and norepinephrine levels were similar between the two groups. Of note, both groups improved treadmill $\dot{V}O_{2max}$ levels; the land-based training group improving 13.8% and the water training group improving 9.2%. Bushman et al. [15] found no significant differences in simulated 5-km runs, submaximal and maximal oxygen consumption, or lactate threshold following 4 weeks of deep-water training in recreationally competitive distance runners.

DISCUSSION

There are several possible explanations for the differences in metabolic response to deep-water running and land-based running. Differences in muscle use and activation patterns contribute to these differences in exercise response. Furthermore, because weight bearing is eliminated and resistance is increased, the larger muscle groups of the lower extremities do less work, and a comparatively increased proportion of work is done by the upper extremities. This may contribute to the lower $\dot{V}O_{2max}$ recorded during deep-water running. Lower perfusion pressures in the legs during immersion, with resultant decreases in total muscle blood flow, also have been proposed to cause a higher anaerobic metabolism during deep-water running [7].

Hydrostatic pressure is thought to assist in cardiac performance by promoting venous return; thus, the heart does not have to beat as fast to maintain cardiac output. This may contribute to the lower heart rates observed during both submaximal and maximal deep-water running. Temperature also has been demonstrated to have an effect on heart rate during exercise, with higher temperatures correlating with higher heart rates.

Familiarity with this form of exercise appears to be an important factor in maximizing physiologic response to deep-water running when measured at a particular level of perceived exertion. In our experience at the Tom Landry Sports Medicine and Research Center and the Houston International Running Center, strict adherence to proper form and technique ensures higher $\dot{V}O_2$ and heart rate.

EXERCISE PRESCRIPTION FOR AQUA RUNNING

Three measures are used for grading aqua running exercise intensity: (1) heart rate, (2) rating of perceived exertion, and (3) cadence. Workout programs typically are designed to reproduce the work the athlete would do on land and to incorporate both long runs and interval-speed training.

Heart Rate

There is a high correlation between heart rate and $\dot{V}O_2$. The American College of Sports Medicine guidelines recommend that for a training effect, exercise should be at a level between 55% and 90% of maximum heart rate (the target heart rate range) [4]. The maximum heart rate can be estimated (220 minus age) or can be based on heart rate levels attained during exercise of maximum effort. Although heart rate levels in the water tend to be lower than on land, it is possible to approach land-based values by adherence to proper technique. Heart rate can be monitored by a waterproof heart rate monitor or periodically by palpation.

Rate of Perceived Exertion

RPE refers to the patient's subjective grading of level of exertion [16,17]. Perceived exertion for jogging is rated as low, whereas sprinting is rated with a high level of perceived exertion. The most commonly used scale of perceived exertion is the Borg

Table 6-2. Borg Scale of Perceived Exertion

Level	Rating of Perceived Exertion
6	
7	Very, very light
8	
9	Very light
10	
11	Light
12	
13	Somewhat hard
14	
15	Hard
16	
17	Very hard
18	
19	Very, very hard
20	

Source: Reprinted with permission from GV Borg. Psychophysical basis of perceived exertion. Med Sci Sports Exerc 1982;14:377.

Table 6-3. Brennan Scale of Perceived Exertion

Level	Rating of Perceived Exertion
1	Very light
2	Light
3	Somewhat hard
4	Hard
5	Very hard

Source: Reprinted with permission from DK Brennan, RP Wilder. Aqua Running: An Instructor's Manual. Houston: Houston International Running Center, 1990.

scale, a 15-point scale with verbal descriptors ranging from very, very light to very, very hard (Table 6-2). The authors use the Brennan scale, a 5-point scale designed exclusively for aqua running; verbal descriptors for this scale range from very light to very hard (Table 6-3) [2]. We further instruct our athletes that level 1 (very light) corresponds to a light jog or recovery run, level 2 (light) to a long steady run, level 3 (somewhat hard) to a 5- to 10-km road pace, level 4 (hard) to 400- to 800-m track speed, and level 5 (very hard) to sprinting (100- to 200-m speed). The Brennan scale facilitates the incorporation of both speed and distance work into workouts in a manner easily understood by both coach and athlete. A sample workout protocol is presented in Figure 6-2.

Cadence

Wilder et al. [18] demonstrated a very high correlation between cadence and heart rate with intraindividual correlations averaging 0.98. Competitive athletes undergo a GXT of aqua running following our standard protocol (Figure 6-3). Cadence is controlled by an auditory metronome. By recording heart rate responses to various levels of cadence,

Workout #1

Total Work- out Time	No. of Repetitions	Duration of Repetitions (min)		Exertion Level		Recovery Periods (sec)
37 min	5	×	2	@	SH	30
	8	×	1	@	H	30
	5	×	2	@	SH	30

Figure 6-2. Sample workout protocol. In this case, the workout protocol calls for five repetitions of 2 minutes' duration each at a perceived exertion level of somewhat hard (SH), followed by eight repetitions of 1 minute's duration each at a perceived exertion level of hard (H), followed by five repetitions of 2 minutes' duration each at a perceived exertion level of somewhat hard, with a 30-second recovery period consisting of easy jogging after each interval, for a total workout time of 37 minutes. (Reprinted with permission from DK Brennan, RP Wilder. Aqua Running: An Instructor's Manual. Houston, TX: Houston International Running Center, 1990.)

we can anticipate an expected physiologic response to a particular cadence level. Workouts then can be designed that use timed intervals at particular cadence levels.

Measurement of heart rate is used primarily during long runs: prolonged periods of exercise at a specified rate (the target heart rate). RPE and cadence ratings are most often used for interval sessions. RPE is most helpful in group settings, whereas cadence is most appropriate for individual sessions.

PRACTICAL GUIDELINES FOR CLINICIANS

Our athletes typically undergo one or two individual sessions for familiarization, to ensure proper technique. A flotation device is used because it is difficult to adhere to proper technique without support. The athletes then undergo our GXT, allowing us to correlate cadence and perceived exertion to heart rate responses. Workouts are then designed using perceived exertion and cadence to effect a particular level of physiologic response. Training schedules are designed to follow closely the work that the athlete would do on land. Thus, for example, if an athlete was scheduled to do six 600-m runs at a pace of 2 minutes each on the track, the athlete would perform six 2-minute intervals in the water at a Brennan perceived exertion level of 4. Longer runs may call for aqua running up to 1–2 hours at a Brennan perceived exertion level 2.

For nonrunners and athletes seeking general conditioning and fitness maintenance only, three to four sessions per week are performed at maintenance duration (15–60 minutes) and intensity (55–90% maximum heart rate). Aqua running is also effectively incorporated into cross-training programs involving other forms of exercise, such as biking and stair-climbing.

As the athlete gradually returns to land-based running, sessions are tapered; however, many athletes choose to incorporate one or two sessions of aqua running per week into their regular training programs.

Name: _____   Date: _____

Predicted 90% maximum heart rate: _____

Stage	End Point	Cadence (gait cycles/min)	Heart Rate	RPE	Comments
W	at 4 min	48			
1	at 6 min	66			
2	at 8 min	69			
3	at 10 min	72			
4	at 12 min	76			
5	at 14 min	80			
6	at 16 min	84			
7	at 18 min	88			
8	at 20 min	92			
9	at 22 min	96			
10	at 24 min	100			
11	at 26 min	104			
Post	at 27 min	48			
	at 28 min	48			
	at 29 min	48			

Figure 6-3. Houston International Running Center Data Collection Sheet: Wilder Graded Exercise Test for Aqua Running. (W = warm-up phase; Post = cool-down phase; RPE = rate of perceived exertion.) (Copyright 1990, Houston International Running Center, Houston, TX.)

AQUA RUNNING FOR SPECIAL POPULATIONS

We have also incorporated aqua running into fitness and rehabilitation programs for nonathletes. These include patients with lumbar spine disorders, arthritis and degenerative joint disease, postoperative orthopedic patients, lower extremity amputees, and women with uncomplicated pregnancies. We emphasize neutral spine mechanics for patients with lumbar spine disease. These mechanics are then incorporated into land-based exercises. Technique is generally modified in patients with arthritis and degenerative joint disease as well as in postoperative orthopedic patients to allow exercise within pain-free ranges. In pregnant women who are unaccustomed to regular exercise, heart rates are maintained under 140 bpm, as recommended by the American College of Obstetricians and Gynecologists [19].

CONCLUSION

Despite the differences between deep-water running and land-based running, deep-water running does elicit the physiologic responses necessary to promote a training effect as defined by the American College of Sports Medicine (40–85% of $\dot{V}O_{2max}$ or 55–90% of maximum heart rate). These responses may be maximized by adherence to proper technique and by the use of environment-specific means of exercise prescription (established specifically for deep-water exercise). Deep-water running also offers additional benefits, most notably the maintenance of quick turnover (rapid gait cycling) as well as coordinated movements between the arms and legs. These aspects facilitate return to land-based training.

Maintaining conditioning is a challenge for the injured athlete. Aqua running is an effective way to continue training during rehabilitation and can later be incorporated into a regular training program, providing a low-stress form of additional cardiovascular exercise.

Further research should help define the effect of aqua running on physiologic parameters other than oxygen use and heart rate as well as responses in special populations. Questions have also been raised regarding differences between shallow-water and deep-water exercise. The increasing interest in aquatic exercise and research will help to answer these questions and expand the use of aquatic exercise for rehabilitation and fitness.

REFERENCES

1. Edlich RF, Towler MA, Goitz RJ, et al. Bioengineering principles of hydrotherapy. J Burn Care Rehabil 1987;8:580.
2. Brennan DK, Wilder RP. Aqua Running: An Instructor's Manual. Houston, TX: Houston International Running Center, 1990.
3. Wilder RP, Brennan DK. Physiologic responses to deep water running in athletes. Sports Med 1993;16:374.
4. American College of Sports Medicine. Guidelines for Graded Exercise Testing and Prescription (4th ed). Philadelphia: Lea & Febiger, 1991.
5. Butts NK, Tucker M, Smith R. Maximal responses to treadmill and deep water running in high school female cross country runners. Res Q Exerc Sports 1991;62:236.
6. Butts NK, Tucker M, Greening C. Physiologic responses to maximal treadmill and deep water running in men and women. Am J Sports Med 1991;19:612.

7. Svedenhag J, Seger J. Running on land and in water: comparative exercise physiology. Med Sci Sports Exerc 1992;24:1155.

8. Town GP, Bradley SS. Maximal metabolic responses of deep and shallow water running in trained runners. Med Sci Sports Exerc 1991;23:238.

9. Bishop PA, Frazier S, Smith J, et al. Physiologic responses to treadmill and water running. Phys Sports Med 1989;17:87.

10. Ritchie SE, Hopkins WG. The intensity of exercise in deep water running. Int J Sports Med 1991;12:27.

11. Yamaji K, Greenly M, Northey DR, et al. Oxygen uptake and heart rate responses to treadmill and deep water running. Can J Sports Sci 1990;15:96.

12. Michaud TJ, Brennan DK, Wilder RP, et al. Aqua running and gains in cardiorespiratory fitness. J Strength Conditioning Res 1995;9:78.

13. Eyestone ED, Fellingham G, George J, et al. Effect of water running and cycling on maximum oxygen consumption and 2-mile run performance. Am J Sports Med 1993;21:41.

14. Wilber RL, Moffat RJ, Scott BE, et al. Influence of water run training on the maintenance of physiological determinants of aerobic performance. Med Sci Sports Exerc 1995;28:1056.

15. Bushman BA, Flynn MG, Andres FF, et al. Effect of four weeks of deep water run training on running performance. Med Sci Sports Exerc (in press).

16. Borg GV. Psychophysical basis of perceived exertion. Med Sci Sports Exerc 1982;14:377.

17. Carlton RL, Rhodes EC. Critical review of the literature on rating scales for perceived exertion. Sports Med 1985;2:198.

18. Wilder RP, Brennan DK, Schotte DE. A standard measure for exercise prescription for aqua running. Am J Sports Med 1993;21:45.

19. American College of Obstetricians and Gynecologists. Exercise During Pregnancy and Postnatal Period Home Exercise Programs. Washington, DC: American College of Obstetricians and Gynecologists, 1985.

7

Asthma and Exercise*

Claudio Gil Soares de Araújo and Oded Bar-Or

Swimming is likely the most universal sport. Individuals of all ages swim for leisure, physical conditioning, or health promotion. More than 100 years ago, swimming for asthma was prescribed for Theodore Roosevelt, and today, it is a common recreational activity and competitive sport for patients with asthma.

There are at least two different aspects of the relationship between exercise and asthma. Training (i.e., regular physical exercise over weeks or longer) is one of the therapeutic modalities for asthma and other chronic respiratory disorders. Acute physical exercise (of several minutes' duration), however, sometimes provokes an asthmatic attack, called *exercise-induced asthma* (EIA). These apparent contraindications often leave practitioners unsure whether to prescribe exercise for their asthmatic patients or recommend that they refrain from intense physical activity.

This chapter reviews the phenomenon of EIA as it relates to aquatic activities (mostly swimming, but also water polo and less-structured water-based games) as well as the benefits of water-based training. First, we provide a brief overview of the epidemiology, pathophysiology, diagnosis, and management of EIA.

EXERCISE-INDUCED ASTHMA

EIA is defined as an asthmatic attack provoked by physical effort. Typically, there is a transient airflow obstruction after intense exercise (in some cases, during exercise) that becomes maximal 5–15 minutes after the activity and is followed by a slower spontaneous return to baseline airflow within 20–90 minutes [1–3].

Epidemiology

EIA can be elicited in most asthmatic patients. Prevalence figures range from 60% to 100% [3–7]. Although all asthmatics develop EIA if they exercise hard enough [8],

---

*Reprinted with permission from CGS de Araújo, O Bar-Or. Asthma, exercise-induced asthma, and aquatic physical activities. J Back Musculoskel Rehabil 1994;4:309.

there is great variability in the day-to-day occurrence of EIA [2]: Although some patients develop asthma almost every time they exercise, others have it only on rare occasions [5]. There is no clear relationship between EIA and the severity of asthma [9]. An isolated clinical picture of EIA in an otherwise healthy individual is rare [10].

Pathophysiology

The pathophysiology of EIA has generated a lot of interest and controversy [3,11,12]. Airway hyper-reactivity seems to be closely linked to EIA [6]. Possible etiologies of EIA include exercise-induced mediator release from mast cells [12] and granulocytes; respiratory heat loss (due to cold inspired air or evaporation of mucosal fluid) [13,14], causing bronchial vascular bed dilation; respiratory water loss, causing increased pulmonary tissue osmolarity [11]; and parasympathetic mediation through vagal innervation [7].

Although water and heat loss from the respiratory tract occur simultaneously, there is some evidence that increased osmolarity caused by water loss is an independent and perhaps the most relevant stimulus for EIA. By manipulating the air temperature, Anderson [11] found that EIA is not always associated with airway cooling. Using a similar approach, Argyros et al. [15] were able to show that mucosal dehydration is the essential pathophysiologic event in the induction of EIA. This mechanism is important in understanding the low asthmogenicity of aquatic sports.

The possible contribution of the parasympathetic nervous system to the mediation of EIA has been studied, with controversial results. Although Tinkelman et al. [16] found that prior inhalation of atropine sulfate blocked EIA in 17 of 18 children, Hartley and Davies [17] concluded that very high doses are necessary to prevent EIA in asthmatic adults. Because children and adolescents have a higher vagal tone compared to adults [18], it is possible that a vagal component would be more relevant for the pathophysiology of EIA in children than in adults. Despite its obvious therapeutic implications, this interesting possibility has yet to be studied.

It is possible that the mechanism of EIA varies among asthmatics, and even in the same patient over time. This would explain the large number of medications that have been found to prevent EIA. In addition to beta$_2$-agonists, cromolyn sodium and ipratropium bromide, alpha-adrenergic blockers [19], leukotriene-D4 receptor antagonists, calcium channel blockers [6], and, most recently, heparin [20] have, in various degrees, produced satisfactory results as EIA blockers.

Diagnosis

To diagnose EIA, one should conduct a standardized 6- to 8-minute exercise provocation test (e.g., on a cycle ergometer, a treadmill, or a step), at a constant intensity that raises heart rate to 85% or more of predicted maximum. In children, heart rate should exceed 160 beats per minute. Some clinicians have been using less standardized conditions (e.g., running up and down a staircase). Although such activities can provoke EIA, their reliability is questionable. A drop of at least 15% (10%, according to some) in forced expiratory volume (FEV) in the first second, or in peak expiratory flow rate, is considered diagnostic [1,3,5,8].

Management

The best management strategy for EIA is prevention. Recently, Brook [6] provided a practical approach to a drug-based treatment of EIA that starts with the use of a beta$_2$-adrenergic agonist inhalant (1 or 2 puffs) 15–20 minutes before exercise. If this is not fully protective, the addition of aerosolized cromolyn sodium is often effective. In selected cases (possibly in patients with a high vagal tone), ipratropium bromide, an anticholinergic inhalant, appears useful. Once EIA occurs, it is easily reversed by bronchodilator inhalants, such as salbutamol (cromolyn sodium is not useful to reverse EIA). On very rare occasions EIA requires more aggressive treatment, or even hospitalization [8].

Prevention or amelioration of EIA can also be achieved by other than pharmacologic means, as per the following recommendations: Perform low- to medium-intensity activities (e.g., those that can be carried out without noticeable hyperpnea) rather than intense activities. The former are less asthmogenic. Adopt aquatic rather than land-based exercise activities. On cold days, put a scarf over the nose and mouth. This helps to humidify and warm the inspired air. For the same reason, use nasal rather than oral breathing whenever possible.

PHYSIOLOGIC RESPONSES TO AQUATIC EXERCISE

Cardiorespiratory responses and adaptations to aquatic exercise, being somewhat different from those observed in land-based exercise, can aid in understanding the benefits of aquatic exercise for asthmatics. A major difference is related to the volume of inspired air. Lower minute ventilation (the volume of air breathed in one minute) is usually found during swimming than during running, for similar intensities of exercise, with no impairment of normal gas exchange [21]. The most remarkable hemodynamic response is a lower maximal heart rate during aquatic exercise compared to land-based activities. This is likely due to a combination of vagal stimulation provoked by facial immersion or diving reflex (i.e., a reflex, vagally mediated bradycardia induced by sudden facial cooling consequent to immersion in cold or ambient-temperature water) and a larger stroke volume caused by the horizontal body position and increased central blood volume.

Swimmers with a prolonged training history often have larger lung volumes and capacities (especially vital capacity). These may reflect an increase in respiratory muscular strength or a more efficient breathing pattern [22]. In addition, pulmonary diffusing capacity both at rest and during exercise is significantly higher in swimmers than in nonswimmers [23,24].

SWIMMING AND ASTHMA

For many years, swimming has been prescribed as a therapeutic activity for asthmatics. It is now common practice to have asthmatic children attend swimming classes or clubs [25]. Even in high-level competitive sports, asthmatics lean toward aquatic events. For example, almost 30% of the members of the Australian swimming team in the 1976 Olympics had asthma [9]. Thus, it is widely recognized that asthma is no longer a barrier to achieving excellence in swimming competition.

Low Asthmogenicity

The main reason for the popularity of aquatic activities among asthmatics is the low asthmogenicity of these activities [1,26–28]. In a classic study, Fitch and Morton [27] compared the presence of EIA after an 8-minute submaximal exercise routine that included running, cycling, and swimming groups. They found that EIA was much less frequent in swimming than in other types of exercise. They also found that in those who respond with EIA to all exercise challenges, smaller declines in FEV were seen after swimming, as compared to running and cycling.

As reviewed by Bar-Or and Inbar [29], various mechanisms have been proposed in an attempt to explain the lower asthmogenicity of swimming. They include the absence of pollen in water, effect of hydrostatic pressure on the chest, hypoventilation, hypercapnia, peripheral vasoconstriction, high humidity of inspired air, horizontal body position, and immersion in water. Most of these factors have not been studied experimentally. Inbar et al. [30] have shown that the prone body position cannot explain the low asthmogenicity of swimming.

There is no definitive answer, but it seems that the most important factor is the high water content of inspired air at water level. Such high humidity prevents the drying and cooling of the respiratory mucosa, in contrast to the drier inspired air during land-based exercise [26,28,29].

Another factor is lung hyperinflation. Although hyperinflation is considered pathologic, it may improve buoyancy and, consequently, swimming efficiency and performance.

Effectiveness of Swim Training as Therapy

Studies by various groups have shown that swim training is beneficial for asthmatics [25,31–36]. Most of these report a reduction in morbidity and an increase in aerobic fitness. Huang et al. performed a well-designed study of the effects of swim training on morbidity [32]: Ninety 6- to 12-year-old schoolchildren with asthma were randomly divided into a control and a training group. The training group was given a 2-month swim training program (three 1-hour sessions per week). Information was then gathered for 12 months and compared with the 12 months that preceded the program. The training group had a 63–89% decrease in the following variables: frequency of attacks, wheezing days, days requiring medication, emergency room visits, rate of hospitalization, and absent school days. The variations in these variables in the control group ranged from 11% to 25%. Peak expiratory flow rate in the training group increased by 63%, compared with 25% in the controls.

In spite of the well-documented reduction in asthma morbidity, there still is debate as to whether swim training results in a decrease in EIA. Svenonius et al. [34] followed 50 children with EIA for 4 months. The children who took part in a swim training program (two 1-hour sessions per week for 3–4 months) significantly increased their working capacity and decreased their degree of EIA. These outcomes are encouraging, but the study did not include a randomly selected control group of patients who did not train, which reduces the validity of the findings. Even when a patient shows a training-induced decrease in the incidence and severity of EIA during daily activities, it is highly likely that EIA would still be elicited if the patient performs high-intensity exercise, especially when large amounts of dry air are ventilated. Notwithstanding, there seems to be a consensus that physically trained asthmatic children will rely less on medications than their untrained peers [8].

In conclusion, considering the scientific data and practical experience, it can be strongly recommended that asthmatic children, and perhaps adults, should participate in regular physical training regimens, with major emphasis on aquatic activities. At least two weekly 30-minute sessions, and ideally five, should be carried out. Aquatic exercise, especially swimming, represents the very first option for individuals of all ages. Even if not mandatory, swimming proficiency is highly desirable and should be strongly recommended. When an individual is unable to swim, water-based games and activities such as "walkaquatics" (walking in the water at various speeds) can be prescribed. One word of caution is necessary regarding scuba diving: Asthmatics should avoid this activity, because a small mucous plug may obstruct an airway, which could then rupture on the diver's return to the surface from a deep dive [37].

PRACTICAL GUIDELINES FOR PHYSICIANS

Most asthmatics benefit from participation in regular aquatic exercise programs. Following these guidelines enhances the likelihood of success:

- Always perform a warm-up routine. It should last more than 3–5 minutes at a low-to-moderate intensity [38,39]. Short sprints are adequate for some asthmatics. Walking in the water or kick-boarding exercises are adequate modes of warm-up. Whenever possible, encourage nasal breathing during warm-up routines.
- Interval training routines (intermittent exercise bouts of 1–3 minutes each) are less likely to induce asthma attacks during exercise than continuous modes of exercise.
- Training intensity should be individually prescribed. Aim not to exceed the person's ventilatory threshold (the intensity at which ventilation increases disproportionately to the increment in exercise intensity) [39].
- There is a higher risk of bronchoconstriction when exercise is performed during the first week after a respiratory infection or within hours after allergen exposure [2,8,40].
- Avoid exposure to air pollution in the pool area, especially sulfur dioxide, black smoke, nitrogen dioxide, and ozone. Some asthmatics are extremely sensitive to these pollutants [41]. High chlorine content may cause airway irritation due to the accumulation of nitrogen bichloride (a derivative of pool chlorine plus sweat or urine). Whenever possible, encourage patients to use outdoor pools (or well-ventilated indoor pools), in which the accumulation of nitrogen bichloride is lower.
- Not all asthmatics are able to enjoy aquatic activities without developing EIA. Those who are prone to EIA should be given 1 or 2 puffs of beta-agonist, inhaled 10–15 minutes before the actual exercise. If this medication is insufficient, sodium cromoglycate could be eventually added by the same route [6]. It is a good idea to ask patients to demonstrate their inhalation technique. Incorrect administration is a common cause of therapeutic failure [42].
- Ascertain compliance to the exercise program. Advise nonregular attendees (and their parents or guardians) of the benefits of a regular aquatic program.

- Regular clinical and laboratory follow-ups account for individual and seasonal variability in asthma. Home peak flow monitoring and daily log reports also seem to be useful [43]. If available, a standardized exercise provocation test should be performed every 6–12 months to confirm the diagnosis of EIA in patients who present with equivocal symptoms. In our experience, negative tests provide an excellent educational experience for patients and parents, who otherwise may continue medication even when it is not needed.

PRACTICAL GUIDELINES FOR PATIENTS AND FAMILY

- Always start exercise sessions slowly and gradually increase the exercise intensity.
- Vary exercise intensities during a single exercise session, avoiding constant-pace exercise.
- Exercise at your own pace; there is no need for or benefit in exercise at maximal intensity.
- Avoid exercise within 1 week of respiratory infection or in the first few hours after allergen exposure.
- If an asthmatic attack occurs with aquatic exercise, it may be useful to have your physician prescribe medications that can prevent recurrence.
- If an inhaled medication has been prescribed, make sure that your use and technique are correct.
- Exercise should be incorporated into your routine; make it a priority. Avoid missing your exercise session.

REFERENCES

1. Bar-Or O. Pediatric sports for the practitioner from physiological principles to clinical implications. New York: Springer-Verlag, 1993;88.
2. McFadden ER Jr. Exercise and asthma. N Engl J Med 1987;317:502.
3. Virant FS. Exercise-induced bronchospasm: epidemiology, pathophysiology, and therapy. Med Sci Sports Exerc 1992;24:851.
4. Kawabori I, Pierson WE, Conquest LL, et al. Incidence of exercise-induced asthma in children. J Allergy Clin Immunol 1976;58:447.
5. Fitch KD, Morton AR. Respiratory Disease. In A Dirix, HG Knuttgen, K Tittel (eds), The Olympic Book of Sports Medicine. Oxford: Blackwell, 1988;531.
6. Brook CJ. Exercise-induced bronchospasm. Postgrad Med 1992;91:155.
7. Mellion MB, Kobayashi RH. Exercise-induced asthma. Am Fam Physician 1992;45:2671.
8. Godfrey S. Exercise- and Hyperventilation-Induced Asthma. In TJH Clark, S Godfrey, TH Lee (eds), Asthma. London: Chapman & Hall, 1992;73.
9. Fitch KD. Swimming Medicine and Asthma. In B Eriksson, B Furberg (eds), Swimming Medicine IV. Baltimore: University Park Press, 1978;16.
10. Konig P, Godfrey S. Prevalence of exercise-induced bronchial lability in families of children with asthma. Arch Dis Child 1973;48:513.
11. Anderson SD. Is there a unifying hypothesis for exercise-induced asthma? J Allergy Clin Immunol 1984;73:660.
12. Broide DH, Eisman S, Ramsdell JW, et al. Airways levels of mast cell-derived mediators in exercise-induced asthma. Am Rev Respir Dis 1990;141:563.
13. Bar-Or O, Neuman I, Dotan R. Effects of dry and humid climates on exercise-induced asthma in children and preadolescents. J Allergy Clin Immunol 1977;60:163.

14. Chen WY, Horton DJ. Heat and water loss from airways and exercise-induced asthma. Respiration 1977;34:305.
15. Argyros GJ, Phillips YY, Rayburn DB, et al. Water loss without heat flux in exercise-induced bronchospasm. Am Rev Respir Dis 1993;147:1419.
16. Tinkelman DG, Cavanaugh MJ, Cooper DM. Inhibition of exercise-induced bronchospasm by atropine. Am Rev Respir Dis 1976;114:87.
17. Hartley JPR, Davies BH. Cholinergic blockade in the prevention of exercise-induced asthma. Thorax 1980;35:680.
18. de Araújo CGS, Nobrega ACL, Castro CLB, et al. Increased cardiac vagal activity in children and adolescents as shown by a 4-s exercise test. Med Sci Sports Exerc 1993;25:S106.
19. Bleecker ER. Cholinergic and neurogenic mechanisms in obstructive airways disease. Am J Med 1986;81(Suppl 5A):93.
20. Ahmed T, Garrigo J, Danta I. Preventing bronchoconstriction in exercise-induced asthma with inhaled heparin. N Engl J Med 1993;329:90.
21. Holmér I, Stein EM, Saltin B, et al. Hemodynamic and respiratory responses compared in swimming and running. J Appl Physiol 1974;37:49.
22. Engstrom I, Eriksson BO, Karlberg P, et al. Preliminary report on the development of lung volumes in young girl swimmers. Acta Paediatr Scand 1971;(Suppl):217.
23. Magel JR, Andersen KL. Pulmonary diffusing capacity and cardiac output in young trained Norwegian swimmers and untrained subjects. Med Sci Sports Exerc 1969;1:131.
24. Yost LJ, Zauner CW, Jaeger MJ. Pulmonary diffusing capacity and physical working capacity in swimmers and non-swimmers during growth. Respiration 1981;42:8.
25. Carlsen KH, Oseid S, Odden H, Mellbye E. The Response of Children With and Without Bronchial Asthma to Heavy Swimming Exercise. In S Oseid, KH Carlsen (eds), Children and Exercise XIII, Vol. 19. Champaign, IL: Human Kinetics, 1989;351.
26. Bar-Yishay E, Gar I, Inbar O, et al. Differences between swimming and running as stimuli for exercise-induced asthma. Eur J Appl Physiol 1982;48:387.
27. Fitch KD, Morton AR. Specificity of exercise in exercise-induced asthma. BMJ 1971;4:577.
28. Inbar O, Dotan R, Dlin RE, et al. Breathing dry or humid air and exercise-induced asthma during swimming. Eur J Appl Physiol 1980;44:43.
29. Bar-Or O, Inbar O. Swimming and asthma—benefits and deleterious effects. Sports Med 1992;14:397.
30. Inbar O, Naiss S, Neuman E, Daskalovich J. The effect of body posture on exercise- and hyperventilation-induced asthma. Chest 1991;100:1229.
31. Fitch KD, Morton AR, Blanksby BA. Effects of swimming training on children with asthma. Arch Dis Child 1976;1:190.
32. Huang SW, Veiga R, Sila U, et al. The effect of swimming in asthmatic children—participants in a swimming program in the city of Baltimore. J Asthma 1989;26:117.
33. Schnall R, Ford P, Gillam I, Landau L. Swimming and dry land exercises in children with asthma. Aust Paediatr J 1982;18:23.
34. Svenonius E, Kautto R, Arborelius Jr M. Improvement after training of children with exercise-induced asthma. Acta Paediatr Scand 1983;72:23.
35. Szentagothal K, Gyene I, Szocska M, Osvath P. Physical exercise program for children with bronchial asthma. Pediatr Pulm 1987;3:166.
36. Tanizaki Y, Komagoe H, Sudo M, Morinaga H. Swimming training in a hot spring pool as therapy for steroid-dependent asthma. Aerugi 1984;33:389.
37. Newhouse MT, Barnes PJ. Conquering Asthma: An Illustrated Guide to Understanding and Care for Adults and Children. Hong Kong: Decker Periodicals, 1991;102.
38. Reiff DB, Choudry NB, Pride NB, et al. The effect of prolonged submaximal warm-up exercise on exercise-induced asthma. Am Rev Respir Dis 1989;139:479.
39. Varray A, Préfaut C. Importance of physical training in asthmatics. J Asthma 1992;29:229.
40. Balfour-Lynn L, Tooley M, Godfrey S. Relationship of exercise-induced asthma to clinical asthma in childhood. Arch Dis Child 1981;56:450.
41. Wardlaw AJ. The role of air pollution in asthma. Clin Exp Allergy 1993;23:81.
42. Charette L. Newer tools for asthma treatment. Mod Med Can 1990;45:854.
43. Stillwell PC. Keeping ahead of childhood asthma. Clin Pediatrics 1993;33:97.

8

Aquatic Therapy:
From Acute Care to Lifestyle

Bruce E. Becker and Juliana Larson

One of the most important qualities of aquatic therapy is its utility across the full spectrum of health care, from the acute management of musculoskeletal injuries to its use as a health-maintaining, physically preserving activity. The physical properties of water provide a margin of therapeutic safety unequaled by most other treatment methods. The opportunity to create a single environment that facilitates both health restoration and maintenance has been left largely undeveloped, however, and most aquatic facilities have specialized in either diseased or healthy populations, but not both. This fragmentation of care divorces disease management from health restoration and rehabilitation as well as from healthy living. As a consequence, the health of the population continues to be impaired by an increasingly sedentary lifestyle, aquatic facilities continue to be underused, and rehabilitative efforts continue to be disconnected and inefficient. This chapter offers a potential solution.

During the late 1800s, preventive and therapeutic health care took place in several distinct venues: hospitals, asylums, sanitaria, and health spas. Patients generally spent little time in hospitals because they were viewed as frightening places generally for the very ill or dying, and convalescence often occurred at home or in sanataria, which usually specialized in a single disease, such as tuberculosis [1]. The healthier segment of the affluent population often used spas for extended recovery and for health maintenance. But during the post–Civil War era, changes in transportation and communication facilitated the development of the general hospital as the primary site of health care, so that from 1873 to 1920, the number of hospitals in America grew from 200 to 6,000 [1].

With the rise in numbers of hospitals, the spa was thought of less as a treatment facility than as a health resort, largely for the affluent. With the advent of widespread antibiotic use, sanitaria began to close. Hospitals occasionally housed pools, but the field of physical therapy was in its infancy. Fear of disease precluded widespread use of pools in most hospitals. Many spas had resident physicians, most trained in European aquatic techniques, but as hospitals became the focus of health care, the spas became more centers of a diverse social life, with promenades, clubs, cotillion, mask balls, and other balls [2]. From the mid-1800s until the early 1900s, hydropathic facilities were built in the major American cities, serving the needs of the public afflicted with chronic illness but rarely those with acute illness. But both spas and urban water cure establishments underwent a significant decline in the early part of this century [2].

The modern whirlpool was developed in Germany at the turn of the century and was used extensively by the French army in World War I. The first one installed in the United States was at Walter Reed Hospital, the U.S. Army facility in Washington, DC. Sidney Licht describes the gradual acceptance of the whirlpool, so that by the time of the end of World War II, nearly every hospital with a therapy department had one. The modern Hubbard tank was first described in 1928, as a device permitting a broader range of exercises, useful particularly in arthritis [2].

In these facilities, patients were almost always treated individually, treatment sessions were short, and the (authorized!) recreational use of these facilities was nonexistent. During the latter half of this century, fewer general hospitals included pools in new construction because of construction and maintenance expenses. Freestanding rehabilitation hospitals nearly always included a therapeutic pool, often using these pools for group classes and activities and sometimes for recreational events for disabled populations but rarely for the general public. At the same time, the community pool was developed largely with the able-bodied individual in mind. Many pools were built with no feasible access for the disabled and had no programming to encourage disabled individuals to use the facility. There was little crossover between the community and the therapeutic aquatic world.

Today, aquatic therapy occurs in many venues. Most aquatherapy still happens in small facility-based pools, under therapist supervision, in one-on-one settings. Many facilities with moderate-sized pools use them for group sessions, often for disease-based populations, such as juvenile arthritis. Occasionally, these facilities serve as a site for community groups but often in a mission-based way, such as a seniors program.

Community pools have rarely had significant linkage with the formal health care system. YMCA pools usually offer the arthritis program that they codeveloped with the Arthritis Foundation. School-based pools frequently offer some group exercise programs, but because of school scheduling, they rarely allow the public during school hours. Programming is fragmented, facilities are underused, and there is poor coordination of programs.

The message that we hope to communicate is that much is to be gained through interfacility coordination and communication. The underpinning value is that a healthy lifestyle needs to combine prevention, occasional rehabilitation, exercise, and education, and that this can happen easily in the aquatic environment.

AQUATIC THERAPY FACILITIES

A broad range of facilities is currently in use in the provision of aquatic therapy. Table 8-1 lists the most frequently used options, their designs, their advantages and disadvantages, and typical programs offered.

The range of facilities is broad. Many communities possess all these options, and among them, there is an aquatic therapeutic venue to suit most patient populations. But the coordination between facilities is often suboptimal, and even awareness of program options elsewhere in the community is poor. With coordination and communication, a patient could move seamlessly from acute management through

Table 8-1. Aquatic Therapy Facilities

Health facility pools
Design
 Typically warm water, 88–94°F (31–34°C)
 Typically 2.5–4.0 ft deep, even bottom or gradual slope
 Often ground level, with access difficult for groups
 Usually small, preventing large group treatment
 Expensive staff (high salaries and wages, trained worker shortage)
 Sling or ramp access most common
Advantages
 Usually medically knowledgeable staff
 Access to health facilities makes acute patient treatment safer
 Warm water more comfortable for low-level activities and prolonged staff immersion
 Ease of access for even severely disabled patients
Limitations
 Limited depth options
 Shortage of trained and experienced staff nationally
 Lack of temperature adjustability precludes some populations, such as patients with
    multiple sclerosis
 Liability requires high level of supervision, typically individual
 Restricted public access is typical
 Ground level makes transfers to and from the water labor intensive
 High temperature restricts use for advanced conditioning activities
Suitable populations
 Hospital-based acute rehabilitation
  Joint replacement, other orthopedic populations
  Neurologic rehabilitation
 Early outpatient
  Arthritis and arthoplasty rehabilitation
  Neurologic rehabilitation
  Rehabilitation programs for deconditioned people
Program and technique options
 Bad Ragaz ring method
 Halliwick method
 Aquatic massage
 Low-level conditioning activities
 Red Cross arthritis classes
 Conventional physical therapy, usually 78–82°F (26–28°C)
Community pools
Design
 Ground level
 Cool water
 Usually ladder or stair access
 Varying depths, typically 3–9 ft
 Heavy occupancy
Advantages
 Public access
 Varying depths make broad range of program options feasible
 Ideal for high-level conditioning programs
 Vertical and horizontal exercise options feasible
 Extended hours often available
Disadvantages
 Staff size limited
 Medical expertise lacking
 Cool water makes low-level activities (e.g., passive aquatic therapies) difficult
 Difficult environment for the severely disabled

Table 8-1. (*continued*)

Program and technique options
    Community open swim programs
    Lap swim programs, including swim teams
    Swim classes
    Limited special population programs usually offered
Hot tubs, spas, and therapeutic tanks
  Design
    Small, low volume
    Single depth, shallow to very shallow
    Hot water, usually ≥101°F (38°C)
    Added turbulence often featured
  Advantages
    High heat level makes low-level activities comfortable
    Heat level therapeutically useful for joint rehabilitation
    Turbulence diminishes pain, may reduce swelling
  Disadvantages
    High heat limits patient populations, treatment length
    Shallow depth limits activity range
    Small size limits activity range
    Essentially individual treatment modality
  Technique options
    Simple range-of-motion exercises
    Joint mobilization
Deep-water environments
  Design: Variable, from diving sections to custom-built facilities
  Advantages
    Permits full gravity off-loading
    Broad range of vertical exercises available
    May range from acute rehabilitation to high-level conditioning
    Swimming skill not required
  Disadvantages
    Require close supervision
    Usually require flotation apparatus
    Fewer staff familiar with possibilities
    Difficult with hydrophobic population
  Technique options
    Aquajogging and water running
    Aqua-dance or ballet movements
    Wide range of aerobic movement options
    Gravity-eliminated range-of-motion exercise

subacute recovery into lifestyle maintenance using each facility at an appropriate time and place. This is an aquatic therapy ideal, too infrequently achieved.

CASE STUDY: PROTOTYPE OF AN IDEA

Eugene, Oregon, is a community of approximately 150,000, served by two major hospitals, and an active Department of Parks and Recreation. In 1987, neither hospital had a therapeutic pool, and although the parks and recreation system had a number of pools, they were not coordinated with the health care system. The Easter

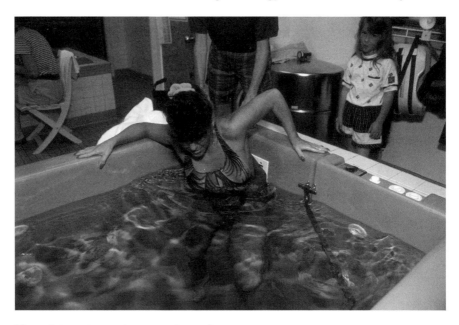

Figure 8-1. Pool entry via wheelchair transfer.

Seals program built a large therapeutic pool with philanthropic dollars, largely for the use of the pediatric disabled population. The authors saw a need for an adult therapeutic pool and approached both hospitals, but at the time neither was interested in investing money and energy in the project. In the autumn of 1987, we decided to begin a program on our own, under the business name of SciEx, Inc.

Space was secured in a medical office building adjacent to the larger of the two hospitals, and facility planning began. The facility was built to include two large, deep-water tanks. These tanks were manufactured by Therapeutic Systems, Inc. (Philadelphia, PA), and were prototypes of the current Aqua-Ark systems. Each tank, 6.5 ft × 5 ft × 6 ft deep, had its own heating system, so that pool temperatures could rapidly be adjusted up or down depending on the patient being treated and the activity. We typically heated them to 88–92°F. Each had its own filtration and chlorinating system. The water treatment and high-turnover filtration was considerably in excess of conventional swimming pool standards. To facilitate transfers into and out of the tank, they were built partially above ground to a lip height equal to that of a seated wheelchair patient (Figure 8-1). The tanks were large enough to accommodate vertical suspension of patients, who were tethered in one to four directions, and supported by flotation devices. The facility included a reception/waiting area, adjacent showering and bathroom facilities, a storage room for pool supplies, and a pool manager's office with full-length sliding glass doors onto the pool area. We negotiated with the hospital for acquisition of a part-time physical therapist, and the facility employed a full-time aquatic therapist, in addition to a part-time exercise physiologist (Figure 8-2).

A thorough evaluation of each patient was made before program entry, including a physician evaluation, present functional capabilities, patient expectations, and outcomes sought. The program incorporated education, attitude adjustments, and motivation. The patient was able to exercise from the first session in a gentle protected

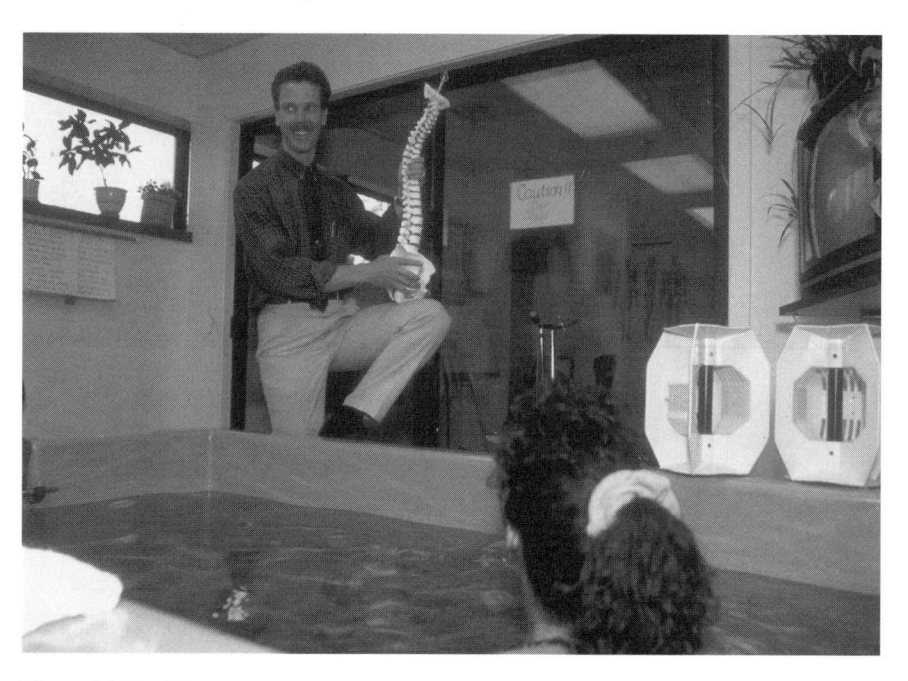

Figure 8-2. Poolside patient education.

motion (depending on ability level) to vigorous movement in a gravity–off-loaded environment. Individual programs were developed for specific musculoskeletal dysfunctions, and individuals were directly supervised during exercise. Constant repetition demonstrated to the physiatrist and the therapist the patient's retention level and skill in maintaining appropriate body posture. This required a coordinated team effort, and communication occurred on a daily basis. The close coordination allowed for modification of goals and treatment plans as necessary.

Patient referrals came with prescriptions that contained the diagnosis, hydrorehabilitation modalities desired, and duration and frequency of treatment. This standard referral was then translated into fluid mechanics, considering the individual's needs and the desired functional outcome. The translation process often required a significant amount of creativity in the choice of specific exercises, equipment, and program of activities. Our services were most commonly requested when conventional physical therapy had failed to achieve the desired functional outcome.

The facility rapidly attracted a broad range of clients, from those with acute athletic injuries, including fractures and stress fractures, to hospital inpatients. Patients with chronic neurologic disease were treated next to elite athletes (Figure 8-3). Workers injured on the job were treated beside Olympic competitors. An aquatic specialist provided clinical oversight under the direct supervision of a physical therapist and a physiatrist. We found through experiment that the ideal treatment length was 45 minutes, and we began to design a structured set of deep-water exercises that could be adapted to the needs of a broad population range. Normal tank temperature was set at 88°F, but we frequently lowered the temperature to 78°F or lower for some multiple sclerosis patients or raised the temperature into the mid-90s for patients in very early treatment phases. Often, we would lower the temperature during the session, so as to prevent core temperature rise during strenuous exercise. We

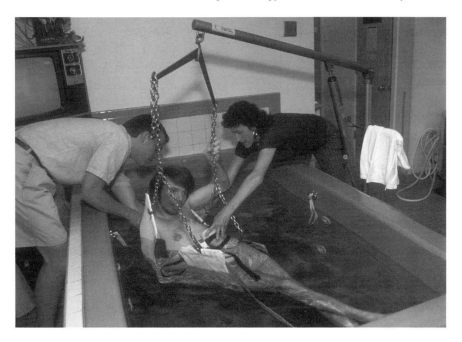

Figure 8-3. Sling transfer of neurologically impaired patient.

found that our most effective marketing tool was word of mouth among the athletic and medical communities. The facility became known within the Department of Parks and Recreation, and we began a series of liaison education sessions with department personnel.

In the beginning, third-party billing was managed in standard fashion, and we typically used the existing pool therapy code, which was at that time CPT 97240 and 97241. Reimbursement was adequate to cover expenses quite early on, and at the first anniversary, the facility was profitable. We spent a considerable time educating third-party case workers and invited many to the facility to watch treatment sessions for covered patients, generally to the satisfaction of the third-party system.

We found that there was no suitable flotation system for high-intensity, deepwater workouts. Consequently, we began the process of designing a belt that would allow tethering, flotation in the appropriately upright position, and adjustment for a range of girths and flotation needs and that would not bind during strenuous workouts. This design was subsequently acquired by Excel Sports Science, Inc. (Eugene, OR) and is currently marketed as the Aqua-Jogger. With this device we found that we could keep even the most muscularly dense elite athlete in proper position. Design changes were constant, even when the device was commercially produced, and we cut out and added foam where appropriate to achieve the desired result (Figure 8-4).

Evolution of Documentation

One of the key elements in the process of third-party billing is documentation. We found that we had to develop our own systems of accountability for progress. We

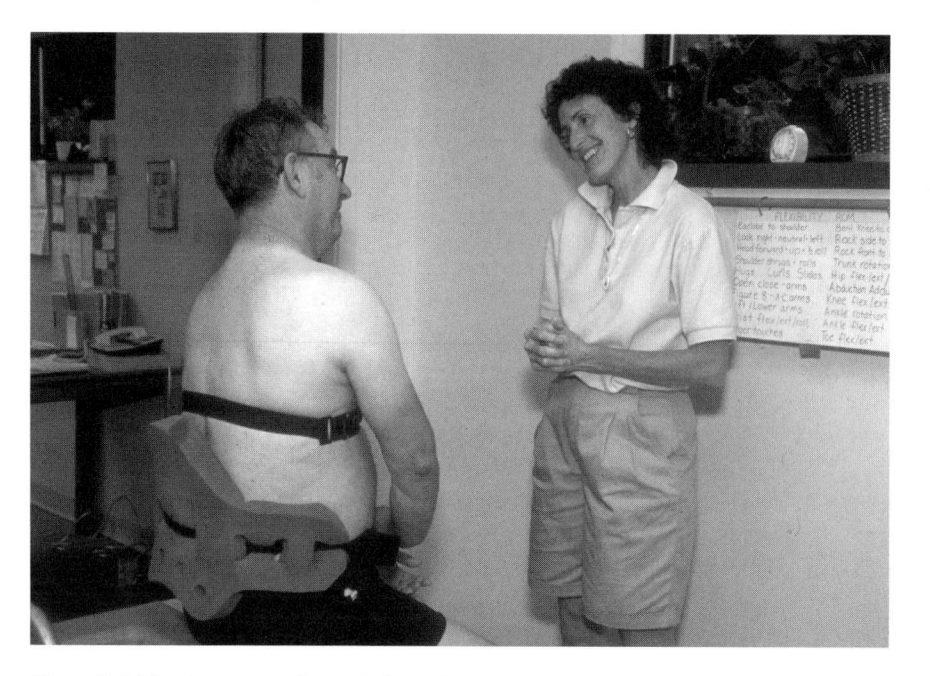

Figure 8-4. Flotation systems for vertical exercise.

could not find a useful initial evaluation format that served our needs, so we created one. It evaluated the individual's medical status, pre-existing medical problems, medications, swimming background, and exercise habits and included a pain disability scoring sheet. From these data, we built an aquatic plan of care. Trial and error showed that an optimal treatment week was two or three sessions; we found no greater objective benefit from four or more sessions per week, and there was significant slowing of rate of gain with one session per week. We listened to the case managers, who expressed a need for refinement of daily visit notes. We began with the system of charting developed by Lawrence Weed (SOAP charting) with sections on subjective aspects, objective aspects, assessment of progress and goals, and plan of care. A formalized protocol was established for each patient treatment session. Programs were structured to generally include at least

- A functional flexibility test before and after treatment
- Monitored perception of pain levels before and after treatment
- Progressive activity levels (1–10), organized into interval set format
- Heart rate monitoring and cadenced music or videos
- Stretching and relaxation exercise by the whirlpool jets

These factors were measured and compiled into a daily patient status log.

We developed a formalized daily note that assessed pain after the previous session, progress on a functional status impairment scale, sleep pattern, new symptoms, measured range of motion and flexibility, and response to exercise with respect to both pulse rate in water and relative perceived exertion during exercise (Figure 8-5). To establish a measurement system for exercise progression and documentation of progress, we developed an endurance workout measurement scale for the program of specific exercises. We asked the patients to monitor their early

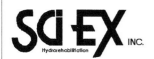 INC.

Hydrorehabilitation Progress Report

Name:_____   Date: _____

Session No: **1** 2 3 4 5 **6** 7 8 9 10 11 **12** 13 14 15 16 17 **18**
19 20 21 22 23 **24** 25 26 27 28 29 **30** 31 32 33 34 35 **36**
37 38 39 40 41 **42** 43 44 45 46 47 **48** 49 50 51 52 53 **54**

SUBJECTIVE REPORTING

Linear Pain Scale: 1 2 3 4 5 6 7 8 9 10
    Pretreatment   _____
    Posttreatment   _____

Response Since Last Session:

Injury Site Tenderness:	Worse	Same	Improved
Muscle Tenderness:	Worse	Same	Improved
Relaxation:	Worse	Same	Improved
Mobility:	Worse	Same	Improved
Energy:	Worse	Same	Improved
Sleep Pattern:	Worse	Same	Improved
Other Therapy:	Worse	Same	Improved
Home Program:	Worse	Same	Improved

Significant complaints/comments:

OBJECTIVE PROGRAM ACTIVITY

	Level	PE	Time	Individual Program
Flexibility/ROM:	____	.__..	____	_____
Strengthening: (Mod. Oxford)	____	.__..	____	_____
Endurance Interval:	____	.__..	____	_____
Relaxation:	____	.__..	____	_____
Pulse Rate:	__ __ __			
Monitored Heart Rate:	____		**Body Wt.:**	**Flexibility:**

Perceived exertion achieved:____

Starting: [   ]   Pretreatment [   ]

Current: [   ]   Posttreatment [   ]

OVERALL ASSESSMENT:

TREATMENT PLAN:

©1990, Sciex, Inc. _____   _____
                 Supervisor   **Therapist**

Figure 8-5. Hydrorehabilitation progress report. (Copyright 1990, SciEx, Inc., Eugene, OR.)

morning pulse rates but with little success. We created a weekly summary report, which was compiled from the day sheets and included objective measurement of progress toward goals, barriers to achievement, range of motion and flexibility, pain levels, endurance testing, and changes in goals and plans. Summaries were sent to referring sources and to insurance carriers for billing purposes.

Next we established a transition program, which we termed *homework*. This usually required that the patient make a visit to one of the community pools and meet with the pool manager to assess program options and times. Early on, we began the process of transferring the patient into the community with a record of his or her program for poolside use and with a log book for review with the patient's treating physician. Our discharge summary format compiled the initial evaluation with the weekly summaries and outcome data. We attempted to compile a record of those patients who continued in pool therapy following discharge to compare with those patients who did not continue, but this proved impossible to achieve reliably through phone contact. Several outcome studies compared functional outcome measures before and after therapy.

There was significant turnover of physical therapists. This led to some inefficiencies because the background and experience in aquatic therapy varied widely among therapists, and our documentation systems had rapidly become quite specific and rigorous. The exercise physiologist departed, but we had incorporated most of the physiologist's guidance into our core program so that there was no major program impact. The hospitals noticed the success of the facility. The smaller hospital built its own therapy pool, and the hospital adjacent to us negotiated with the Easter Seals program to allow an expanded outpatient adult population to use the facility. Several community-based physical therapists negotiated with local health clubs for pool use time. None of these other programs actively sought linkage with the broader community Parks and Recreation program, though, so we did have an advantage with case managers.

The Parks and Recreation connection had become quite deep by the end of 1991, and as a result, many of our protocols could be readily transferred to the community. We found the relationship with the department to be symbiotic because they could more readily defend their budget by explaining the ties with the health care system, which required slightly higher staffing ratios and more complex programming. In late 1992, SciEx closed its doors as the first author moved to Michigan and the second author joined the Department of Parks and Recreation as Director of Sheldon Pool Programs.

ANOTHER CASE STUDY: THE IDEAL PROCESS

One of the most important lessons learned from our experience is the potential importance of a community support system for hospital-based aquatic therapy activity. Such a program serves the needs of the patient while lowering health care costs, encouraging patient responsibility, and building a base of individuals sufficient to support unique program needs.

Integration of programming into a broad range of population needs is demonstrated in the concept of the Aquatic Hub (Figure 8-6). The mission of Hub programs is to provide progressive levels and options of aquatic activity in a comfortable, familiar, caring, and educational environment. The Aquatic Hub bridges the gap between hospital-based therapy programs and an active exercising

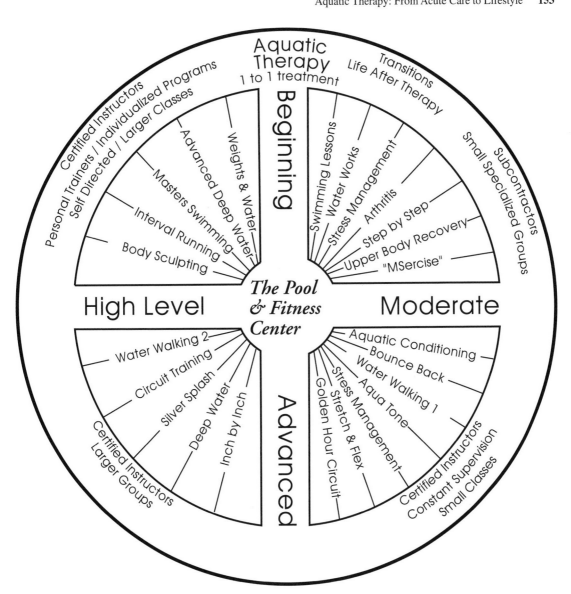

Figure 8-6. The Aquatic Hub. Interdisciplinary approaches to progressive aquatic programming. Community pools meeting the continuum of needs from the physically challenged to the physically fit. (Copyright 1993, revised 1995, Juliana Larson, B.S., L.M.T., and Sylvia Schepps, C.R.T.)

lifestyle. By using the "learning moment" provided by an injury or illness and initiating an aquatic exercise regimen when appropriate, the patient becomes aware of the usefulness of aquatic therapy in recovery. By moving the patient early into the community setting, while the willingness to alter lifestyle is still present, the individual gains familiarity with the community pool environment. Once the patient is involved, the Hub's diverse programming fulfills the patient's expectations of competent instruction through individualized classes and fitness choices. This truly

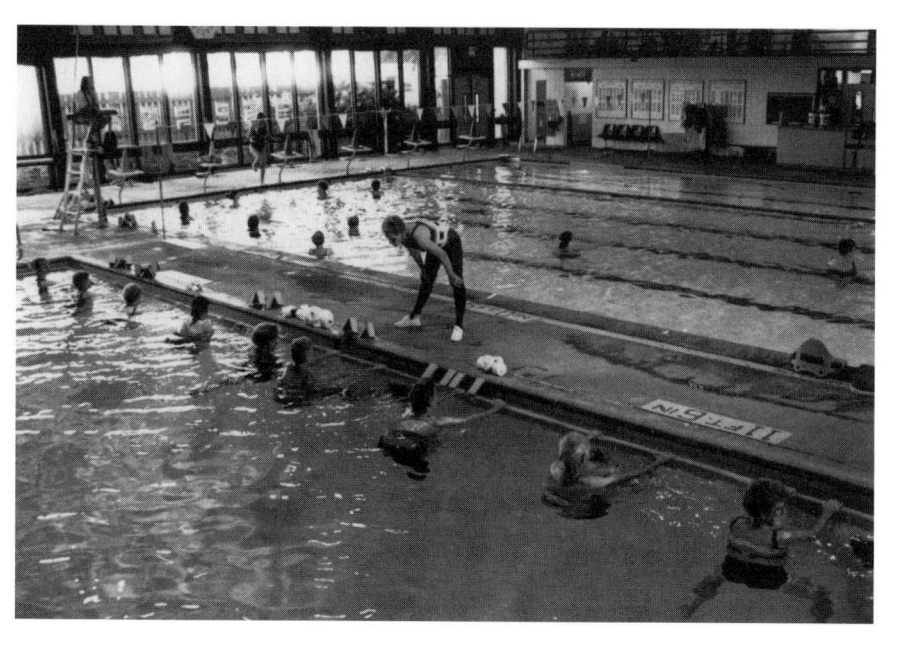

Figure 8-7. Pool overview at Sheldon Pool and Fitness Center. (Copyright 1996, Susan Detroy, Eugene, OR.)

benefits the mission of municipal facilities to provide a range of structured, supervised classes to benefit the broad taxpayer base. The Aquatic Hub is a management and citizenry effort to maximize the use of the facility and staff with the goal of promoting wellness. This concept is achieving great success at Sheldon Pool and Fitness Center in Eugene, Oregon.

Sheldon Pool is one of eight year-round pools in the Eugene-Springfield metropolitan area, serving a population of 150,000. Sheldon has two rectangular pools, one a 25-yd, six-lane, graduated-bottom pool and the other a diving well (Figure 8-7). Both pools are maintained at 85.5°F. The pools are convenient to parking, wheelchair accessible (Figure 8-8), and attractive.

It is the goal of the Sheldon staff to structure a program for any individual to maintain or improve the function he or she has gained from therapy or to continue to enhance recreational opportunities the individual wants to pursue. In this facility's programming, a patron can receive the continuum of care needed after therapy to continue on a recovery pathway. The staff works with the individual to assist in achieving the skill and knowledge to continue from life after therapy to a fitness level that meets his or her daily and recreational needs. It is a challenge to the staff to design a sufficient variety of classes to meet the needs of all patients, from top athletes to the severely physically challenged. Experts from many disciplines participate, including a massage therapist who teaches back conditioning classes, athletic trainers and marathoners who teach deep-water running classes, a midwife teaching pre- and postnatal classes, a movement therapist teaching stress-release stretching classes, and an oncology nurse or mastectomy patient teaching upper body recovery classes. The pool encourages community therapists to contract pool time to run small-group or individual sessions with patients next to swim classes or water fitness classes to which a patient may move when ready. Programs beget

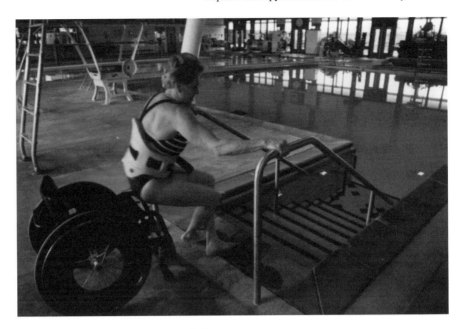

Figure 8-8. Entry access for limited ambulators.

more programs, and teachers emerge from the group of pupils, so the process is a dynamic, vital one. The challenge is to have a director with the skills to recruit teachers, schedule programs, plan with the general and health communities, and negotiate the tricky waters of the municipal budget process. All these classes began on paper, were presented to the public, and are being well attended at Sheldon Pool, along with the more traditional classes for arthritis, multiple sclerosis, aquatoning, seniors, and beginning through advanced deep-water classes. At present, the pool runs 72 water-fitness classes per week and 148 swim lessons, including all American Red Cross levels plus infant, adult, and adapted programs (Figure 8-9). Every day, the facility hosts 12 hours of child care, 4 hours of after-school activity, and 4 hours of recreational swimming; each week there are two to four community meetings and 4–10 hours of massage therapy. Temporary employees account for 87% of personnel, which lowers staffing costs.

It is important that the community pool, as the center of the Aquatic Hub activities, be a drawing point for all ages and ability levels, serving as a learning facility for swimming as a life skill, a meeting place for support groups as well as team sports, and a satellite for physical, occupational, and recreational therapy. The Hub should promote an intergenerational approach to lifelong fitness. The patrons, clients, patients, health care providers, and insurance companies that refer should trust the facility management to be responsive to their needs. The communication and educational processes should go both ways.

The intent of the program is to provide sufficient options so that no reasonable need is unmet. The availability of on-site child care removes one major obstacle. The wealth of class opportunities removes another. Physical accessibility removes an important obstacle to the transition process for disabled people. There should be no screening for acceptability, as is the case in many health clubs. Ideally, an interdis-

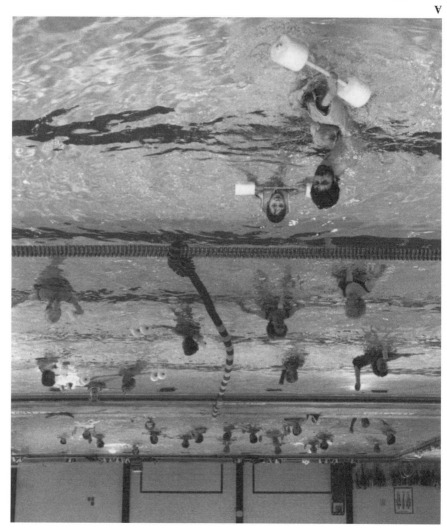

A

Figure 8-9. A. Simultaneous classes in operation. B. Different generations performing different activities simultaneously. (Copyright 1996, Susan Detroy, Eugene, OR.)

ciplinary program of this type promotes multigenerational usage for a diverse community. Within the same block of time, a grandmother, a daughter, and a grandson should be able to participate in different enjoyable and therapeutic activities under the same roof. The results of this creative programming include staff loyalty and enthusiasm, high customer service and satisfaction, increased attendance, and community support.

It is significant that the Eugene-Springfield area is one of the most penetrated areas in the nation with respect to managed care. Consequently, area physicians are constantly searching for practical methods of decreasing health care costs without compromising health care quality. Sheldon Pool plays an increasingly important role in this effort: It is often used as a primary therapy resource, either through involvement with a therapist working with one of our programs or by direct recommendation of a patient to one of our programs. Physicians encourage patients to

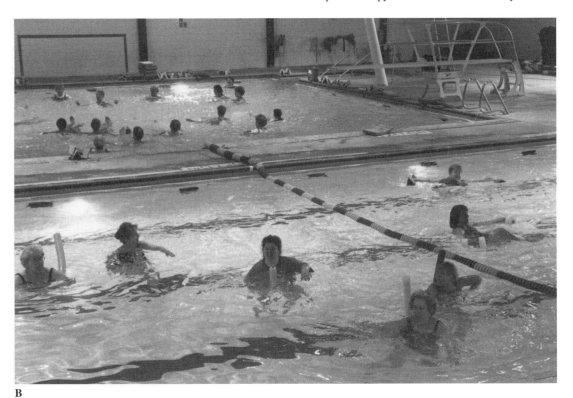

B

move from formal hospital-based therapy activities into one of our programs, which require fewer therapy sessions and encourage more responsibility on the patient's part. For aquatic therapy to be cost-effective, though, it must be efficient and facility use must be high because maintenance and upkeep costs are great, even for small facilities.

One of the by-products of the Americans with Disabilities Act of 1994 is the requirement for all public recreational facilities to become fully accessible. Consequently, it is now feasible to develop larger subspecialized programs for disabled Americans with unique needs and to meet these requirements in community facilities. Accessibility creates a larger market opportunity. In the past, the disabled community has had limited access to fitness facilities, and deconditioning-related health care consequences are common. Community facilities such as Sheldon Pool open avenues to healthier lifestyles for this population, but every community facility now has the opportunity to better serve their community as well. Although it is true that accessibility improves life for the disabled, it also benefits parents with strollers, older adults with grandchildren in tow, and many others.

Barriers and Facilitators

The success of the Sheldon Pool is largely due to the efforts and energies of many people within the Department of Parks and Recreation to the support of the broad external community, particularly health care providers. It has also taken many years and much dialogue to break down the barriers of suspicion, professional jealousy, and competition over turf. To start, a key barrier was the attitude that a community pool facility is an inappropriate site for health care activities. For physicians to develop trust in the facility, a great deal of communication was necessary. Program development had to respond to suggestions from the provider community, and patient outcomes needed to reflect follow-through. A significant advance in credibility was made when physical therapists began to create programs within the facility. It is difficult to assess the impact that the managed care environment had in building willingness in the health care system to release a patient from a more costly service to a potentially less costly one. Another barrier was the physical distance between the facility and any health care facilities.

The difficulty of finding trained program leaders, especially in new areas, also presented problems. We have found that innovation has enabled us to work our way through this problem: Using movement therapists, oncology nurses, nurse midwives, and others has actually become a strength. However, not every step along the way has been smooth.

A significant barrier is the complexity of coordinating all these programs. Although multidisciplinary programming sounds ideal, rescheduled or misbooked classes have offended many. Open communication mends some of these wounds, but some participants leave, never to return. The goal is to replace them with flexible, open class leaders.

The traditionalism of the health care community has at times been a barrier. There is almost no substantive outcome research in aquatic therapy, so it is simply impossible to reassure physicians that there is a body of research supporting some of our programs. Here again, the managed care environment has facilitated openness to new and alternate methods. Eugene-Springfield has always had a strong untraditional element in its population, so a traditional attitude has presented more professional concerns than public ones. The public must always know that professionalism prevails, however, and this requires that programs must be clinically solid and respectable. Traditional programs may be created in innovative ways. Nontraditional programs must be created around traditional values: personal responsibility, integrity, and ethical standards of care.

CONCLUSION

Traditional health care has taken place largely within formal medical environments. Although it serves to isolate the person who is ill, this division from society has not facilitated change. The health care system is now changing radically. Public recognition of the value of exercise is widespread, even if the practice is not. As a society we are becoming more obese and more sedentary, and we are spending more on health care costs associated with these issues. Yet often, community aquatic facilities are underused, and even more often they are isolated from any contact or involvement with the health care system.

A potential solution may be moving health maintenance and prevention out of the health care facilities and into the community. Lifestyles built around healthy exercise, socialization across generations, and development of a sense of community are likely to improve more than the public health status: They may begin the process of healing society. This may sound like too grand a goal for aquatic therapy, but with a broad regional effort, the creative juices of many individuals, and the collaboration of a diverse group of involved professional and community leaders, it is possible to make a significant start. In so doing, the health and well-being of many and the benefit of the community will be served. We hope that our example may serve as a springboard for many more beneficial facilities.

REFERENCES

1. Starr P. The Social Transformation of American Medicine. New York: Basic Books, 1982;76.
2. Kamenetz HL. History of American Spas and Hydrotherapy. In S Licht (ed), Medical Hydrology. New Haven, CT: Elizabeth Licht, 1963;160.

9

Risk-Management Strategies for the Therapy Pool*

Marilou Moschetti and Andrew J. Cole

To prevent minor and major accidents, employees and owners who provide therapy services in the aquatic environment must do risk-management planning. It is essential that patients and staff be familiar with regulations, codes, operations, maintenance, contraindications, and appropriate measures for personal safety in and around the therapy pool.

This chapter defines the relationship between risk management and aquatic therapists, delineates the areas of risk in aquatic therapy environments, and provides recommendations for basic risk management in aquatic therapy environments.

DEFINING RISK MANAGEMENT AND ITS RELATIONSHIP WITH AQUATIC THERAPY

Risk management is the practice of assessing risks inherent in a program or facility and attempting to eliminate or minimize them through implementation of change [1].

Managing risk is necessary to prevent accidents in aquatic settings. This is especially important in places or during activities that may be hazardous to human health and safety. Many health hazards are associated with exercise in the aquatic environment, including an inadequate knowledge of personal safety and insufficient swimming skills. If an aquatic therapist hopes to provide a safe and efficiently run facility for patients, special care and attention must be given to developing and maintaining high standards and practices of risk management.

SPECIFIC PROBLEMS AND AREAS OF CONCERN FOR PATIENT SAFETY

Drowning is the number one risk in an aquatic environment. The American Red Cross [2] identifies the three most prevalent causes of drowning in pools: (1) failure

---

*This article has been adapted with permission from ML Moschetti, AJ Cole. Aquatics: risk management strategies for the therapy pool. J Back Musculoskel Rehabil 1994;4:265.

to recognize hazardous conditions and practices, (2) inability to get out of dangerous situations, and (3) lack of knowledge about the safest ways to aid a drowning person. All can be prevented by training in basic water safety skills. Use of alcohol and drugs, diving into shallow or unknown water, overestimating physical ability and stamina, and medical emergencies in or around bodies of water, are the most common causes of drowning [3]. For safe swimming, therapy pools must have nonslip surfaces, an emergency communication system, water-depth markings, and a lifeguard on duty. The staff must be trained in personal water safety measures, such as breath control and bobbing, floating on the back, survival floating, treading water, and releasing a cramp. Simple safe-reaching techniques are basic methods of water rescue (Table 9-1).

There can also be problems with maintenance, such as water sanitation and handling of chemicals and equipment. Unexpected environmental emergencies, such as earthquakes, gas leaks, power outages, and floods, can occur [4]. During an earthquake, light fixtures and other building parts can fall into a pool and cause injury or electrocution. Power outages and floods create emergency evacuation problems, especially when the pool is located in the basement of a building. Gas leaks can cause respiratory emergencies for patients and staff [5]. To minimize the risks they pose, these situations must be anticipated and plans must be made.

When oxidizing and sanitizing agents are inadequate, a buildup of bacteria in the therapy pool can create infectious conditions [6]. High bather loads and careless water-testing procedures can also lead to increases in bacteria. Pathogens in human feces are the main culprits (Table 9-2).

Risk of illness depends on time spent in the water, skin hydration with altered skin flora, and toxic reaction to enzymes or endotoxins produced by a specific bacterium [7–10]. Pool water must be laboratory tested on a regular basis. The Environmental Protection Agency's (EPA) Safe Drinking Water Hotline (800-426-4791) provides a list of certified water-testing laboratories. (See the chapter appendix for additional resources.)

Exposure to endotoxins (airborne particles from the cell walls of dead bacteria) can create respiratory problems in the enclosed therapy pool. The Solar Energy Research Institute, Harvard Medical School, and the National Centers for Disease Control have conducted research on endotoxin conditions. In 1989, a rare respiratory condition, hypersensitivity pneumonitis, was diagnosed in two lifeguards in Westminster, Colorado; the pool was closed because of endotoxin proliferation. Closure was attributed specifically to the sanitizing agents used in facility operations. Consequently, a retrofit of circulation and mechanical-room equipment, with ozone as the primary sanitizer, was performed and the problem was solved [11,12].

Exposure to blood-borne pathogens is another risk that must be managed by aquatic therapy facility staff and owners. The Occupational Safety and Health Administration (OSHA) says that fire and first-responder personnel are exposed to hepatitis B approximately 8,700 times a year, and about 200 die as a result. An exposure is defined as a situation where transmission from an infected person can take place, that is, there is a carrying agent, an active carrier, and a susceptible recipient [13]. An exposure may involve the mouth, eyes, other mucous membranes, or nonintact skin, and it may involve contact with blood or other potentially infectious materials. A patient's fall on a pool deck or in a facility's dressing room may lead to exposure for aquatic personnel. Lifeguards and other people exposed daily to potential carriers must be trained to deal with environmental hazards they may encounter on the job [14].

Table 9-1. Safety Procedures in and Around the Therapy Pool

Safety rules and procedures for staff and patients

No inflatable tubes, air mattresses, or artificial supports (e.g., flotation belts) should be substituted for swimming ability.

Never allow anyone to enter pool without staff present.

Avoid long periods of immersion in hot water baths, hot tubs, or spas where water temperature affects heart rate and respiration.

Emergency exits must be clearly marked in pool area and dressing rooms. An emergency communications system must be available in dressing rooms.

Emergency evacuation equipment must be kept on the pool deck and inspected regularly. Necessary equipment includes a shepherd's crook, life ring, rescue tube, resuscitation apparatus, spine board, blanket, and scissors to cut off equipment.

Keep a well-stocked first-aid kit on or near the pool deck.

Keep a list of pool users' telephone and combination lock numbers in case of emergency. Personal belongings may need to be returned or removed and nearest relatives contacted.

Means of entering pool by stairs, ramps, or ladders should be appropriate for patients' ambulatory abilities. Provide a lift for nonambulatory patients.

Keep all pool decking and dressing areas free of excess water.

Benches, chairs, and toilet seats in the dressing room should conform to code, be the correct height for patients, and be in good working order at all times.

Provide adequate ventilation in the dressing rooms.

Avoid electric shock by eliminating hair dryers where water may be present in the dressing rooms.

Emergency water extraction (partial list of procedures)

Identify patient's position: vertical, prone, or supine. Choose a method to open the airway, and identify flotation or breathing equipment that must be removed from the patient.

Outline the procedures to follow for each type of drowning: passively floating or actively thrashing.

Prepare for evacuation; have emergency equipment ready.

All aquatic personnel must know their responsibilities: Who calls 911? Who evacuates the patient? Who directs pre- and post-EMT response?

A diagram of the pool is used to identify the exact location for the response team. The team has knowledge of the site and can gain access to it immediately on arrival.

Unlock exit doors and notify the administration office.

Documentation of the accident should be completed immediately after the accident, the insurance company must be notified, and all information must be kept on file for the life of the facility.

Aquatic personnel in-service training and documentation

Each staff person should be able to perform safe-reaching rescue techniques. A safe-reaching rescue allows the rescuer to safely extend his or her reach beyond the pool edge. This technique is usually used with the rescuer in a prone or stable position. Specific techniques include the use of a rolled towel, rescue tube, shepherd's crook, or other object for the victim to grasp.

Staff training should occur regularly. Conduct simulated emergencies to test and evaluate response systems for individual and group situations every 3 months. All typical emergency scenarios should be documented in the employee procedures manual.

Emergency telephone 911 system, security cameras, and direct voice communications to administration from pool area should be provided during operational hours.

A log of in-service training dates, type of training, and personnel present must be kept on file for insurance purposes (at least 5 years).

Each staff person should learn to use a rescue technique called *head-chin support* and head splint for immobilizing the cervical spine.

An inspection log of the facility's maintenance room, dressing rooms, pool area, use of chemicals, cleaning schedule, and all other health and safety regulations must be kept on file at all times.

If a gas chlorinating system is in use, identification of mechanical room's emergency response hazard system should conform to all health and safety codes for local and state guidelines.

If a child is hurt, records of the accident must be kept on file in the facility office until the child reaches age 18½.

Sources: A Osinski. The complete aquatic guide. Parks & Rec 1990;25(2):36; The American Red Cross. Swimming and Diving. St. Louis: Mosby–Year Book, 1992;23; Department of Health Services. The Design, Construction, Operation and Maintenance of Public Swimming Pools. In California Administrative Code. Sacramento, CA: Department of Health Services, 1986; AJ Cole, RE Eagleston, ML Moschetti. Swimming. In AH White (ed), Spine Care, Vol 1. St. Louis: Mosby, 1995;727; and A Osinski. Risk management issues for aquatic physical therapy. Orthop Phys Ther Clin North Am 1994;3(4):111.

Table 9-2. Causes of Infectious Conditions in Therapy Pools

Agent	Means of Transmission and Condition
Intestinal (coliform) bacterium	Enters the body through cuts and abrasions
Giardia lamblia	Infection by a protozoan cyst which is transmitted by fecal discharge, causing diarrhea
Pseudomonas aeruginosa	Swimmer's ear and folliculitis
Staphylococcal bacterium	Skin boils
Cryptosporidium	Causes prolonged diarrhea and cramps; spread by egglike particles in animal feces; resistant to chlorine
Chlamydia bacterium	Swimming pool conjunctivitis, an eye infection spread by genital secretions

Under the guidance of the Centers for Disease Control, universal precautions have been developed for controlling occupational exposures to hepatitis B, human immunodeficiency virus (HIV), and other potentially infectious materials. Because of water's chemical and physical properties, viral particles apparently cannot be transmitted through pool water, even without the presence of chlorine or other halogens. Personal protective equipment, written work-practice controls, and staff training help to prevent exposure to blood-borne pathogens while performing job duties [15–17].

BASIC REGULATIONS AND CODES GOVERNING AQUATIC FACILITIES

State and federal codes and regulations govern all aquatic facilities where human health and safety are potentially at risk [18]. Such codes and regulations are generic and not uniform across states. They are referred to as *state bathing codes*, and violations are considered misdemeanors punishable by fines. The codes cover physical plant sites, maintenance-room equipment, water-sanitizing materials, and all elements of safety for pool users and staff [19]. Some codes overlap, but the major guidelines and public laws that regulate how pools operate are standard throughout the swimming pool industry.

OSHA Occupational Exposure to Blood-Borne Pathogens Control Plan 29 CFR 1910.1030

This plan is designed to reduce employees' risk of exposure to pathogens such as fungi, germs, bacteria, hepatitis B, and HIV. Lifeguards and other aquatic personnel may come into contact with human blood or other body fluids during certain procedures and equipment use. Personnel who have a high probability of exposure must be given a pre-exposure hepatitis B vaccine at no cost.

U.S. EPA, Superfund Amendments Reauthorization Act Title III: Emergency Planning and Community Right-to-Know Act

This act requires facilities to report hazardous material storage, obtain permits for use, and provide inventory and maps for each site where the material is used. Chlorine is such a material. Data on reportable quantities of hazardous substances spilled or released into the environment must be reported by telephone and by written report to the EPA.

U.S. EPA–Department of Agriculture Pesticide Worker Safety Regulations

Chlorine and other halogens are considered pesticides. A pesticide is a substance or mixture of substances that can be produced economically in large batches and is intended for use in preventing the spread of, destroying, repelling, or mitigating fungi, bacteria, or any other form of plant or animal life declared to be a pest. Training is required for employees who apply or mix antimicrobial products and who maintain, service, or clean contaminated equipment. Canisters of the material require appropriate labeling with EPA registration numbers [20,21].

U.S. Department of Labor OSHA Hazard Communication Standards 29 CFR 1910.1200

Employers must inform employees of hazardous materials and provide the safety equipment needed for protection. This regulation applies to all hazardous materials, including sanitizing agents used on flooring and decking around swimming pools. The document ensures evaluation and communication to prevent and minimize exposures to hazardous substances produced in or imported by the United States. Exposure records, which must be maintained for 2 years, include date of application, location, commodity used, and name of antimicrobial agent. It is also necessary to post Material Safety Data sheets, which are used to inventory all hazardous substances at a facility. All storage containers for antimicrobial agents must be labeled appropriately.

Written Employee Injury and Illness Prevention Program b3203(a)(2) (Where There Is No Labor Union)

This program is used to train employees who are at daily risk of exposure to hazardous materials. Training must be provided when product labeling requires respiratory protection. Employers must provide emergency medical care, labels, washing stations, and safety equipment in locations where hazardous chemicals are used. The cost of lost workdays due to aquatic staff injuries can be reduced by having a prevention program in place.

Uniform Fire Code, Article 80, Hazardous Materials

This code stipulates that when there is storage and maintenance of chlorine gas, local fire district regulations apply and must be followed.

Americans with Disabilities Act (ADA), PL 101-336

The ADA mandates that "no individual be discriminated against on the basis of disability in the full and equal enjoyment of the goods, services, facilities, privileges, advantages, or accommodation by any person who owns, leases (or leases to), or operates a place of public accommodation [s.302 (a)]." The ADA applies to employers with 25 or more employees and requires public accommodations in facilities designed and constructed after January 26, 1993. The ADA lists hotels and motels; places of exhibition, entertainment, and recreation; professional offices of health care providers; parks or places of recreation; schools; social service center establishments; and gymnasiums, health spas, or other places of exercise. Barrier-free access to pools and spas located at these facilities is required. Failure of aquatic-facility owners and employers to comply with the ADA can result in liability due to negligence [22,23].

RECOMMENDATIONS AND CONCLUDING REMARKS

Aquatic therapy is increasingly used as a method of treatment for patients with musculoskeletal, neurologic, and other conditions [24–34]. More than 2,500 facilities in the United States presently provide aquatic therapy services. Hospitals, private-practice therapists, and other providers are constructing pools to accommodate patient needs.

Given the tremendous interest and increase in aquatic therapy, it is surprising that water safety issues may not be addressed during training periods for therapists or physicians. Anyone in an aquatic environment has the potential to drown; therefore, basic water safety skills are of utmost importance in therapeutic settings. Basic principles and policies should be part of any facility (Table 9-3).

Appropriate supervision in and around the therapy pool means having a certified lifeguard (over age 18) on duty during operating hours [35]. Facilities hiring people under age 18 must remember that such employees are not of legal age. Although the individuals may be eligible because they have taken and passed courses certifying them to perform lifeguard duties, they cannot legally be held responsible for their actions. The minimal recommended certifications for aquatic therapy personnel are (1) community water safety, (2) basic first aid, and (3) cardiopulmonary resuscitation. If the therapy pool is located in a very small community and emergency medical services are not available by calling 911, one staff member should be certified in emergency medical treatment. Employees must receive training in universal precautions for emergency medicine. Ideally, at least one member of the staff should be certified by a nationally recognized training agency as a lifeguard and water safety instructor. It is recommended that one staff person take a Certified Pool Operators course offered by a reputable aquatic consultant, company, or provider. The course provides information on engineering controls for the maintenance and management of sanitizing agents, circulation and recirculating equipment, and general pool operation.

Risk management must include professional safety training, and the aquatic staff must learn how to handle difficulties that patients may have and emergencies in and around the pool (Tables 9-4 and 9-5).

Safety in an aquatic environment hinges on adherence to rules designed to protect patients and staff from potential hazards. The development of formal personnel policies and procedures, pool facility operations and management guidelines, emergency and nonemergency communication standards, and documentation are the first steps in pool facility management. Specifically, management policies should include documentation and implementation of (1) standards of conduct with respect to liability, (2) confidential medical questionnaires to be completed by patients, (3) contraindications to pool therapy, (4) safety rules and regulations for patients, (5) emergency water-extraction procedures, and (6) staff training, including personnel rescue and training scenarios (Figure 9-1; see also Table 9-1).

Table 9-3. Aquatic Management Principles, Policies, and Procedures

Each facility establishes conduct standards with respect to liability. Medical intake, prescriptions, informed consent, risk assumption, and general release forms must be part of the procedures manual.

Pool regulations; visible signs identifying water depth, chemical storage, and emergency phone; locker room schematic; and deck equipment must be described or listed in the manual, posted in the pool area and administration office, and filed with the insurance company.

Insurance policies, progress notes, accident and incident forms, and compliance with local, state, and federal health and safety codes must be included in the manual.

Patients sign waiver, release, and indemnity agreements before treatment.

In-service training is documented and a log is kept with participant names, dates, and type of training.

Accident and incident reports are used to identify actions taken by staff, the procedures followed, emergency medical technician response and treatment, and witness and follow-up information.

Patients must sign general pool rules before beginning therapy. Rules include equipment use, bathing suit requirements, drug or alcohol use, lost-and-found policies, diving regulations, deck safety, spa use, showering pre- and post-treatment, and staff supervision requirements.

Confidential medical questionnaire and statement

Patients sign questionnaire to identify heart disease, respiratory problems, muscular conditions, medication, swimming abilities, or other conditions that may alter the response to aquatic therapy.

A medication list is made to identify drugs that might affect participation in therapy. Special note must be made of beta blockers, which could affect a patient's perceived exertion.

Absolute contraindications for patients referred to aquatic therapy [36]

Cardiac failure

Urinary infections

Open wounds or contagious skin rash (draining boils)

Infectious diseases; must be a channel of transmission: conjunctivitis, primary (draining) herpes, airborne

Uncontrolled bowel or bladder incontinence

Vomiting

Scabies or lice

Severe burns

Menstruation without internal protection

Premature rupture of membranes in pregnancy

Suprapubic catheter

Nontunnel catheters: High risk for serious infection (peripherally inserted; single, double, or triple lumen)

Precautions for aquatic therapy (concerns are aesthetic rather than clinical) [36–39]

Hypersensitivity to any sanitizing agents or chemicals used in pool

Thermoregulatory problems

Excessive fear of water

Severely weakened or deconditioned state

Compromised respiratory function and vital capacities

Multiple sclerosis: Water temperature above 88°F may cause fatigue and stress

Perforated eardrum

Ostomy (evaluate for odor, discoloration; empty the collection pouch before pool session)

Intravenous lines: Cover with a transport dressing (Tegaderm) and plastic bag. Tunnel catheters are acceptable following individual assessment (e.g., Hickman/Broviac; Groshong; implanted access device [Port-A-Cath])

Peripheral vascular disease

Incipient cardiac failure

Dysphagia

Epilepsy

Unstable high or low blood pressure

Fever

Inability to enter the pool on one's own can also create a hazard. If transfer equipment is unavailable and the staff-to-patient ratio is low, then additional precautions and staff safety must be evaluated.

Sources: A Osinski. The complete aquatic guide. Parks & Rec 1990;25(2):36; The American Red Cross. Swimming and Diving. St. Louis: Mosby–Year Book, 1992;23; AJ Cole, RE Eagleston, ML Moschetti. Swimming. In AH White (ed), Spine Care, Vol 1. St. Louis: Mosby, 1995;727; A Osinski. Risk management issues for aquatic physical therapy. Orthop Phys Ther Clin North Am 1994;3(4):111; ML Moschetti, AJ Cole. Aquatics: risk management strategies for the therapy pool. J Back Musculoskel Rehabil 1994;4:265; and AJ Cole, ML Moschetti, RE Eagleston. Spine pain: aquatic rehabilitation strategies. J Back Musculoskel Rehabil 1994;4:273.

Table 9-4. Patient Problems

Discomfort or inability to swim (with or without a flotation support) in deep water
Physical fatigue
Respiratory distress
Muscular conditions (e.g., cramps)
Choking

Table 9-5. Emergencies That Staff Must Be Prepared to Handle

Obstructed airway
Severe bleeding
Cardiac conditions, including cardiac arrest and myocardial infarction
Cervical or lumbar spine injury
Seizure
Heat- or cold-related emergencies
Diabetic shock or coma
Broken bones
Electric shock
Vision impairment
Hearing impairment
Fainting

Policies and procedures outline the rights and duties of patients and staff, express the philosophy of the facility, and describe the rationale for programs that are offered. Primary consideration should be given to prevention of accidents and illnesses associated with the aquatic therapy environment. Adequate methods of problem identification, safety evaluation, and careful documentation of daily operations will make facilities safe, pleasing, and therapeutic environments for patients and staff.

Acknowledgment

The authors wish to thank Clint Moschetti for editing a portion of the manuscript.

Facility: _____   Date completed: _____

Yes	No	
☐	☐	**Deck:** Floors are clean and free of water, meet minimum friction coefficients, have no collecting pools of water, and equipment does not block passage.
☐	☐	**Ventilation:** There are no irritating fumes; allowable humidity levels; air turnover rate is acceptable; there is a temperature variance of 5–7°F between water and air; no noticeable drafts are present.
☐	☐	**Lighting:** All lights are operational and tested monthly; the pool's surface is free of glare so that it does not interfere with the lifeguard's ability to see users.
☐	☐	**Water temperature:** Water is maintained at an acceptable temperature for all users and for all activities offered.
☐	☐	**Water quality:** Water quality is within acceptable chemical ranges and is tested every 2 or 3 hours. All drains are visible to the pool bottom; the test kit is kept stocked with fresh reagents, and records are kept of daily analysis.
☐	☐	**Safety equipment:** Rescue tubes, ring buoys, extension poles, first-aid kit, and air horn are all within easy reach and immediately available. All spine boards, cervical collars, and immobilizers are free of defects, placed in appropriate positions, and in good working order; ladders and rails are secured.
☐	☐	**Telephone:** Emergency telephone is available on the pool deck; emergency information is posted next to the phone, including location, street numbers, schematic drawing showing evacuation exits. Pool exercise equipment is stored so as not to impede disabled users or emergency personnel.
☐	☐	**Depth markings:** Pool depth is plainly and clearly marked at and above water surface. Depth is marked in feet and inches, in letters larger than 4 in., and in contrasting colors, such as red and black. Drop-off lines indicate changes in pool slope.
☐	☐	**Signs:** Warning signs are positioned for users to see when entering the therapy pool area (all safety warnings, written and verbal, should be conveyed and understood by users before entering the water); certain signs are required by code and are necessary to convey information that might alter users' behavior in and around the pool.
☐	☐	**Pool rules:** Pool rules are posted clearly for all users of the facility.
☐	☐	**License:** Permit to operate the pool is posted in a conspicuous place.
☐	☐	**Security:** Adequate barriers, alarms, and other security devices are installed, operational, and tested monthly.
☐	☐	**Mechanical room, sanitizing regulations, and general maintenance:** Opening and closing procedures are completed daily. Documentation and training procedure manuals are posted in conspicuous locations. Sanitizing chemicals on decks and in locker rooms and mechanical rooms are stored, labeled, and handled according to hazardous materials specifications. Material Safety Data Sheets are posted. Auxiliary rooms are clean, sanitized, and free of barriers. Emergency-drench showers, safety gear, and eyewashes are available for all personnel handling chemicals.
☐	☐	**Aquatic personnel:** Personnel are dressed appropriately for their duties; lifeguard supervision is adequate for the number of users present; current certifications or licenses are filed in administration office. Staff training is adequate for facility programs and services; training manuals that include job responsibilities and duties, methods of enforcement, emergency plans, and dress codes are in place; staff in-service meetings are held and documented periodically.
☐	☐	**Facility:** The facility complies with all local, state, and federal bathing codes, as well as hazardous materials, OSHA, and other health and safety regulations.

Figure 9-1. Sample inspection checklist for the therapy pool. (Adapted from A Osinski. The Complete Aquatic Guide. Parks & Rec 1990;25[2]:36. References 1, 2, 13, 25, 33 were also used in compiling this list.)

REFERENCES

1. Osinski A. The complete aquatic guide. Parks & Rec 1990;25(2):36.
2. The American Red Cross. Swimming and Diving. St. Louis: Mosby–Year Book, 1992;23.
3. Ellis AA, Trent RB. Hospitalizations for near drowning in California: incidence and costs. Am J Public Health 1995;85:1115.
4. Martinez TT, Long C. Explosion risk from swimming pool chlorinators and review of chlorine toxicity. J Toxicol Clin Toxicol 1995;33:349.
5. Penny P. Swimming pool wheezing. BMJ 1983;5:461.
6. Highsmith AK, Kaylor BM, Calhoun MT. Microbiology of therapeutic water. Clin Manage 1991;11:34.
7. Sharp D. Tainted water. USA Weekend 1996;Jan 5–7;22.
8. Aggazzotti G, Fantuzzi G, Righi E, Predieri G. Environmental and biological monitoring of chloroform in indoor swimming pools. J Chromatogr A 1995;710:181.
9. Favero MS. Problems and solutions. Postgrad Med 1986;80:282.
10. Hollyoak V, Body P, Freeman R. Whirlpool baths in nursing homes: use, maintenance, and contamination with *Pseudomonas aeruginosa*. Commun Dis Rep CDR Rev 1995;5:R102.
11. Matthews-Sargeant PJ. Swimming with the enemy. Pool & Spa News 1993;32(5):42.
12. Herman E. A mystery solved? Pool & Spa News 1993;32(14):20.
13. Collopy C. Aquatic Center Safety Manual: Blood-Borne Pathogens Supplement. San Jose, CA: Environmental Health & Safety Department, San Jose State University, 1992.
14. Kozlowski JC. OSHA cites ocean lifeguarding and mouth-to-mouth resuscitation as risk activities. NRPA Aquatic Newsletter 1992;May:9.
15. OSHA. Bloodborne Facts: Hepatitis B Vaccination—Protection for You. Washington, DC: OSHA Publications, 1992.
16. County of Santa Cruz. Procedures for evaluating exposure incidents. Santa Cruz, CA: Health Services Agency, 1992.
17. OSHA. Hepatitis B Vaccination—Protection for You. Washington, DC: OSHA Publications, 1993.
18. Osinski A. Complying with codes. Athletic Business 1994;18(3):35.
19. Department of Health Services. The Design, Construction, Operation and Maintenance of Public Swimming Pools. In California Administrative Code. Sacramento, CA: Department of Health Services, 1986.
20. OSHA. Hazardous Waste Operations and Emergency Response (29 CFR 1910.120). Washington, DC: U.S. Congress, 1992.
21. County of Santa Cruz. Regulation of the Use of Pesticides, Definitions, Label Requirements, and Codes. Santa Cruz, CA: Agricultural Commissioner Weights & Measures, 1992.
22. Osinski A. Modifying public swimming pools to comply with provisions of the Americans with Disabilities Act. Palaestra 1993;Summer:13.
23. U.S. Department of Justice. Americans with Disabilities Act. Washington, DC: U.S. Congress, 1992.
24. Cole AJ, Eagleston RA, Moschetti ML. Swimming. In AH White (ed), Spine Care, Vol 1. St. Louis: Mosby, 1995;727.
25. Osinski A. Risk management issues for aquatic physical therapy. Orthop Phys Ther Clin North Am 1994;3(4):111.
26. Moschetti ML, Cole AJ. Aquatics: risk management strategies for the therapy pool. J Back Musculoskel Rehabil 1994;4:265.
27. Hurley R, Turner C. Neurology and aquatic therapy. Clin Manage 1991;11:26.
28. Triggs M. Orthopedic aquatic therapy. Clin Manage 1991;11:30.
29. Cole AJ, Moschetti ML, Eagleston RA. Getting backs in the swim. Rehabil Manage 1992;5(5):62.
30. Cole AJ, Eagleston RA, Moschetti ML. Aquatic rehabilitation for the lumbar spine. Your Patient Fitness 1994;8:19.
31. Cole AJ, Moschetti ML, Eagleston RA. Spine pain: aquatic rehabilitation strategies. J Back Musculoskel Rehabil 1994;4:273.

32. Cole AJ, Moschetti ML, Eagleston RA. Lumbar Spine Aquatic Rehabilitation: A Sports Medicine Approach. In DC Tollison (ed), The Handbook of Pain Management (2nd ed). Baltimore: Williams & Wilkins, 1994;386.

33. Cole AJ, Campbell DR, Berson D, et al. Swimming. In RG Watkins (ed), The Spine in Sports. St. Louis: Mosby, 1996;362.

34. Moschetti ML. Facility Design. In R Ruoti, D Morris, AJ Cole (eds), Aquatic Rehabilitation. Philadelphia: Lippincott, 1997;355.

35. Moschetti ML. Aquatic therapy: procedures and strategies for therapists. Presented at the Saint Joseph's Hospital Aquatic Therapy Symposium, Marshfield, WI. April 1993.

36. Shanda LD. Physiological responses to therapy in water. Presented at the annual meeting of the Aquatic Therapy & Rehabilitation Institute, Aquatic Therapy Symposium, Minneapolis, MN. October 1993.

37. Nguyn ND, Wadley HN, Edlich RF. Corrosion of stainless steel pipes in a hydrotherapy pool by a silver-copper disinfection system. J Burn Care Rehabil 1995;16:280.

38. Cammann K, Hubner K. Trihalomethane concentrations in swimmers' and bath attendants' blood and urine after swimming or working in indoor swimming pools. Arch Environ Health 1995;50:61.

39. Decker WJ. Chlorine poisoning at the swimming pool: an overlooked hazard. J Toxicol Clin Toxicol 1978;13:377.

Appendix 9.1

Resources for Aquatics, Swimming Pool Codes, and Regulations

Besides these organizations, check local telephone directories.

American Red Cross
8111 Gatehouse Road
Falls Church, VA 22041
(703) 206-6000

Americans with Disabilities Act
U.S. Department of Justice
Civil Rights Division
P.O. Box 66118
Washington, DC 20035

Aquatics for Special Populations
YMCA Program Store
Box 5077
Champaign, IL 61820
(217) 351-5077

Centers for Disease Control
U.S. Department of Health &
   Human Services
1600 Clifton Road
Atlanta, GA 30333
(404) 639-2317

**International Association
   of Aquatic Consultants**
2417 E. Sheffield Circle
Fort Collins, CO 80526

National Spa & Pool Institute
2111 Eisenhower Avenue
Alexandria, VA 22314

National Swimming Pool Foundation
10803 Gulfdale, Suite 300
San Antonio, TX 78216

OSHA Publication Office
200 Constitution Avenue, NW
Room N-3101
Washington, DC 20210

**U.S. Environmental
   Protection Agency**
Waterside Mall
401 M Street, NW
Washington, DC 20044
(202) 260-4700

10

Overview of Nonswimming Aquatic Research and Rehabilitation

Richard G. Ruoti and Jill Napoletan Craig

With the increasing interest in aquatic exercise and rehabilitation, the need to justify treatment increases concomitantly. Many studies have been performed on swimming and the physiologic response to swimming. Less well documented, however, is the effect of nonswimming aquatic exercise, such as water calisthenics and water running, usually performed in a vertical position. Objective, well-controlled experimental research on therapeutic techniques is grossly inadequate. This chapter presents an overview of the research on the physiologic parameters of nonswimming exercise.

TEMPERATURE

A few studies have investigated temperature as a variable in aquatic exercise. In 1967, Costill et al. [1,2] performed two studies that examined the effect of water temperature on submaximal exercise and aerobic work capacity. Six water temperatures were used, ranging from 17.2°C to 32.78°C. A small group of subjects used an underwater ergometer for various tests. Despite the huge temperature variation, no significant alteration of aerobic capacity was observed in the different water temperatures. Almost a decade later, McArdle et al. [3,4] examined the effect of temperatures at 18°C, 25°C, and 33°C. Six male subjects participated in the study, and oxygen consumption ($\dot{V}O_2$), cardiac output, stroke volume, and heart rate (HR) were measured. The study found no significant difference between $\dot{V}O_2$ in air and in the 33°C water temperature, but significantly higher $\dot{V}O_2$ values were recorded during submaximal work in 18°C and 25°C water. McArdle and his colleagues concluded that the high oxygen cost in colder water was primarily "due to energy expended by shivering as an attempt to maintain core temperature" [3]. They further concluded that working in warmer water demonstrated responses similar to those of subjects working on land. Although these early studies were not training studies, they do suggest that metabolic responses can be elicited in water. The McArdle group study reported increased responses at higher temperatures.

In 1989, Gleim and Nicholas [5] also demonstrated that the higher water temperatures commonly used in hydrotherapy produce an increased HR response in relation to $\dot{V}O_2$. Water heated to 36.1°C elicited higher HR than 30.5°C water, and both varied significantly from HR recorded during similar exercise in 26°C ambient air. These results suggest that the thermal stimulus to increase HR may over-ride the stimulus of immersion to shift the blood centrally and depress the HR.

Whether due to the physical constraints of the pool or to anecdotal information, some researchers have held temperature constant while investigating other variables, such as depth, strengthening effects, $\dot{V}O_2$, and HR.

DEPTH

The Gleim and Nicholas study also manipulated water depth, demonstrating an interaction between depth and temperature. Water temperature appears not to affect cardiac output at levels below the subject's waist.

Napoletan and Hicks [6] found that treadmill running in chest-deep water (32°C) elicited $\dot{V}O_2$ values similar to land-based treadmill running; however, midthigh levels resulted in significantly higher oxygen consumption.

Harrison et al. [7] quantified the amount of body weight relieved by buoyancy relative to the level of immersion. This study also demonstrated that, as intensity of exercise increases, the amount of weight relief at a given depth decreases.

STRENGTH

Increases in strength are not expected in aerobic exercise. It is sometimes reported, however, that water calisthenics increase strength. The literature is sparse in this area and limited to specific populations.

Gehlsen et al. [8] measured muscular strength and endurance of patients with multiple sclerosis after they had completed an aquatic fitness program. The training involved some swimming strokes but also included water calisthenics. Postexercise testing revealed upper-extremity strength improvements, but lower-extremity strength improvements were limited to knee extensors. Likewise, McGettigan and Ruoti studied the effects of a water exercise program on an elderly population. Strength testing of the lower extremities indicated results similar to Gehlsen's. Subjects demonstrated a significant increase in knee extensor strength, but no difference was found for knee flexors [9].

Although Henker et al. [10] demonstrated that water running is effective in maintaining leg strength in runners, Hamer and Morton [11] found no significant change on scores obtained for a 2-minute fatigue test after an 8-week study involving running in 1-m–deep water.

OXYGEN CONSUMPTION

Probably one of the most extensively researched variables in aquatic exercise deals with submaximal and maximal $\dot{V}O_2$. Most physiologists consider $\dot{V}O_{2max}$ to be one of the best overall measurements of physical fitness.

Numerous studies [1–3,5–6,10–19] have examined the effect of aquatic exercise on $\dot{V}O_{2max}$ or have used $\dot{V}O_2$ when correlating other variables. Although some studies were single-bout activities, others were training studies ranging in length from 8 to 12 weeks. These studies consistently demonstrated that $\dot{V}O_{2max}$ increases with training or in a water environment, provided that sufficient intensity, duration, and frequency parameters are met. It was also determined that the $\dot{V}O_2$ and HR increase linearly during submaximal activity, which is consistent with results obtained with exercise on land. These results were achieved after various types of water activity, including calisthenics, walking, running, running while performing an upper body activity, and running with buoyant assistive devices.

As noted, many studies were single-bout activities and therefore did not demonstrate a training effect. Training studies did show, however, increases in $\dot{V}O_2$ as high as 16%, again demonstrating values comparable to those [17] obtained with land-based training.

HEART RATE

HR has been studied or monitored by virtually every physiologic aquatic study cited [18,20]. Some looked specifically at HR in water versus on land. Because it is difficult to quantify work in two different environments, physiologic measurements are used to determine if the work performed is comparable.

Studies using single-bout aquatic activities have consistently demonstrated elevated HR comparable to HR achieved with similarly imposed stresses on land. Likewise, training studies have demonstrated significant increases in work with lower submaximal HR and lower resting HR at the conclusion of the training. These data are important because most people participating in aquatic exercise and rehabilitation programs do not have the luxury of undergoing a monitored stress test. Therefore, HR could be an effective way to prescribe exercise that is both safe and of sufficient intensity to cause a training effect.

REHABILITATION

The clinical use of nonswimming aquatic exercise has increased dramatically throughout this decade. A body of research investigating aquatic rehabilitation has begun to accumulate, supported largely by practitioners seeking to document its efficacy for a given diagnosis or to define and quantify treatment variables.

Several studies have focused on orthopedic conditions of the lower extremities. Tovin et al. [21] reported that patients who underwent an aquatic therapy protocol for anterior cruciate ligament reconstruction displayed less joint effusion and elicited more favorable subjective outcome scores than did patients in a traditional therapy group. In a similarly designed study [22], it was concluded that underwater treadmill ambulation was a beneficial additive therapy for the reacquisition of quadriceps strength and range of motion at the knee.

The water depth study by Harrison et al. [7] is another example of research conducted for practical application to rehabilitation: By quantifying the amount of body weight relieved at different levels of immersion, a progressive weight-bearing protocol could be formulated for the aquatic patient.

DISCUSSION

The research dealing specifically with temperature and nonswimming activity is limited. Nevertheless, most of the studies that demonstrated positive effects [5,7,8,11,13–15,20,23,24] controlled water temperature in the range of 26–30°C (average = 28.64°C). Therapeutic pools that tend to have higher temperatures may be more effective for rehabilitation application, but there are few temperature-controlled studies dealing with patient populations, and therefore a conclusion is not warranted based on current available data. It does appear, however, that if exercise is performed at a sufficient intensity and duration, the effect of temperature in the 26–30°C range is not as critical. Generally, $\dot{V}O_{2max}$ is either increased or maintained with aquatic exercise. Although some studies demonstrate gains comparable to those in land-based activity, others do not. Nonetheless, most show significant improvement to warrant aquatic activity as a stimulus for $\dot{V}O_2$ improvement. The variety of exercises used to promote $\dot{V}O_2$ improvement includes adaptations of familiar land-based calisthenics, aerobic dance movements, water walking, jogging, bobbing, running, and modified swim strokes.

The use of HR for exercise prescription for water-based exercise remains controversial. Some authors [4] have suggested using a lower age-predicted HR when prescribing water exercise; other research studies do not support reduction. Perhaps the answer lies in separating horizontal from vertical exercise, as well as depth of water. Swimming involves greater use of the upper extremities, whereas nonswimming exercise includes more lower extremity involvement. Changes in stroke volume may occur with horizontal positioning, but hydrostatic forces may also influence stroke volume via centralization of peripheral blood flow and increased left ventricular end-diastolic volume. Likewise, immersion depth appears to be influential in HR depending on whether the heart is submerged or not. Research has shown that cardiovascular adjustments are made with aquatic exercise, but a precise prescription for intensity remains elusive.

CONCLUSION

A review of the literature allows the following conclusions:

1. Aquatic exercise can be performed in a wide range of temperatures, but warmer temperatures appear to be more favorable for nonswimming activity.
2. Some studies demonstrated an increase in $\dot{V}O_{2max}$ in water compared to land activities, but others did not. All studies reviewed, however, indicated that significant increases in $\dot{V}O_{2max}$ can occur with exercise in water.
3. After adequate conditioning, resting HR decreases to values comparable to a training bradycardia resulting from terrestrial training, and HR elevates sufficiently to cause cardiovascular conditioning similar to land-based activity.
4. Upper body strength can increase in deconditioned people, but lower extremity strength gains appear to be limited to leg extensors.
5. Given the proper parameters of an exercise prescription of warm-up, intensity, duration, frequency, mode of training, and cool down, nonswimming water exercise can produce a training effect.

RECOMMENDATIONS

Most of the research reviewed here involves healthy populations. Studies have been performed with cardiac patients that have included both swimming and nonswimming aquatic exercise. Current research with patient populations includes studies in orthopedics and pediatrics, but this is not enough.

The majority of articles reviewed have dealt with nonswimming aquatic exercise. Swimming, however, often plays a significant role in exercise training. Therefore, the effects of nonswimming aquatic rehabilitation, the effects of swimming-oriented rehabilitation programs, and a combination of both forms of activity need to be elucidated.

Considerable research is needed to justify treatment not only to patients and insurance carriers, but equally important, to the profession.

Specific questions about exercise prescription, HR, and water temperature need to be answered. It is incumbent on rehabilitation professionals to evaluate and attempt to determine in some way the validity of our efforts with studies involving patients with a variety of diagnoses.

Although aquatic physical therapy protocols for a broad spectrum of diagnoses have yet to be compiled, physicians can feel confident in referring their patients to skilled aquatic physical therapists for rehabilitation. Based on current research, a variety of populations would benefit from the cardiovascular effects and musculoskeletal strengthening and conditioning afforded by aquatic exercise. Cardiac, obstetric, neurologic, orthopedic, spinal cord–injured, and pediatric aquatic rehabilitation protocols need to be developed, researched, and quantified.

REFERENCES

1. Costill D, Cahill PJ, Eddy D. Metabolic response to submaximal exercise in three water temperatures. J Appl Physiol 1967;22:638.
2. Costill D. Effects of water temperature on aerobic work capacity. Res Q 1967;39:67.
3. McArdle W, Magel J, Lesmes GR, Pechar GS. Metabolic and cardiovascular adjustment to work in air and water at 18, 25 and 33 degrees C. J Appl Physiol 1976;40:85.
4. McArdle WD, Katch FI, Katch VL. Exercise Physiology, Energy, Nutrition and Human Performance. Philadelphia: Lea & Febiger, 1991.
5. Gleim G, Nicholas J. Metabolic cost and heart rate responses to treadmill walking in water at different depths and temperatures. Am J Sports Med 1989;17:248.
6. Napoletan J, Hicks R. The metabolic effects of underwater treadmill exercise at two depths. Aquatic Phys Ther Rep 1995;3:9.
7. Harrison R, Hillman M, Bulstrode S. Loading of the lower limb when walking partially immersed. Physiotherapy 1992;78:163.
8. Gehlsen GM, Grigsby S, Winant D. The effects of an aquatic fitness program on the muscular strength and endurance of patients with multiple sclerosis. Phys Ther 1984;64:653.
9. McGettigan J, Ruoti RG. Unpublished thesis. Biokinetics Research Laboratory, Temple University, Philadelphia, 1990.
10. Henker L, Provast-Craig M, Sestili P, et al. Water running and the maintenance of maximum oxygen consumption and leg strength in runners. Med Sci Sports Exerc 1991;24(Suppl):3.
11. Hamer PW, Morton AR. Water-running: training effects and specificity of aerobic, anaerobic and muscular parameters following an eight-week interval training programme. Aust J Sci Med Sport 1990;21:13.
12. Evans FW, Cureton KJ, Purvis JW. Metabolic and circulatory responses to walking and jogging in water. Res Q 1978;49:442.

13. Kirby RL, Sacamano JT, Balch DE, et al. Oxygen consumption during exercise in a heated pool. Arch Phys Med Rehab 1984;1:21.
14. Bishop PA, Frazier J, Smith H, et al. Physiologic responses to treadmill and water running. Phys Sports Med 1989;17:87.
15. Heberlein T, Perez H, Wygand J, et al. The metabolic cost of high impact aerobics and hydro-aerobic exercise in middle aged females. Med Sci Sports Exerc 1987;19(Suppl):2.
16. Fernhall B, Manfredi T, Congdon K. Prescribing water-based exercise from treadmill and arm ergometry in cardiac patients. Med Sci Sports Exerc 1992;24:139.
17. Johnson LB, Stromme SB, Adamczyk JW, et al. Comparison of oxygen uptake and heart rate during exercises on land and in water. Phys Ther 1977;57:273.
18. Cassady SL, Nielsen DH. Cardiorespiratory responses of health subjects to calisthenics performed on land versus in water. Phys Ther 1992;17:532.
19. Ruoti RG, Troup JT, Berger RA. The effects of non-swimming water exercises on older adults. J Orthop Sports Phys Ther 1994;19:140.
20. Michaud T, Brennan D, Wilder R, et al. Aquarun training and changes in treadmill running maximal oxygen consumption. Med Sci Sports Exerc 1991;24(Suppl):5.
21. Tovin B, Wolf S, Greenfield B, et al. Comparison of the effects of exercise in water and on land on the rehabilitation of patients with intra-articular anterior cruciate ligament reconstructions. Phys Ther 1994;74:710.
22. Napoletan J. The effect of underwater treadmill exercise in rehabilitation of surgical anterior cruciate ligament reconstruction [unpublished Master's thesis]. Orange, CA: Chapman University, 1991.
23. Vickery S, Cureton K, Langstaff J. Heart rate and energy expenditure during aquatic dynamics. Phys Sports Med 1983;11:67.
24. Whitley JD, Schoene LL. Comparison of heart rate responses: water walking vs. treadmill walking. Phys Ther 1987;67:1501.

Index

Date Due

2/27/98			
APR 0 3 1999			
JUL 0 6 2000			
FEB 2 7 2003			
MAR 1 9 2003			
NOV 2 8 2003			
DEC 0 1 2006			